# PRIMAL PLATES

## Mastering a Meat-First Lifestyle for Sustainable Health and Lasting Vitality.

# Dr. Lucy J. Patrick

# Copyright Page

*Primal Plates: Mastering a Meat-First Lifestyle for Sustainable Health and Lasting Vitality*

**Copyright © Dr. Lucy J. Patrick**
**All rights reserved.**



**Disclaimer**

This book provides information on a meat-first dietary approach for general wellness and vitality, grounded in the author's research and professional experience. *Primal Plates: Mastering a Meat-First Lifestyle for Sustainable Health and Lasting Vitality* is intended solely for informational purposes and is not a substitute for medical advice. Readers should consult a healthcare professional before making any dietary, exercise, or lifestyle changes to ensure suitability based on their individual health needs.

The author and publisher disclaim any liability for direct or indirect effects arising from the use of information presented in this book. All dietary, exercise, and supplementation recommendations are general and may not be appropriate for all readers. Readers are encouraged to make informed decisions and seek personalized guidance from qualified health practitioners where necessary.

# Table of content

Incorporating natural supplements into a meat-based diet can improve performance, recovery, and overall health, particularly for those seeking fitness. 137

# Introduction

The Rise of the Primal Plate Lifestyle

The Primal Plate lifestyle emphasizes a meat-first approach, focusing on high-quality animal products while minimizing carbohydrates. This diet promotes health benefits such as weight loss and reduced inflammation, contrasting with more restrictive diets like vegans or paleo. Misconceptions about meat consumption often stem from outdated beliefs; however, studies show that a meat-based diet can enhance overall well-being. The "Primal Plate" concept encourages a balanced intake of meats, healthy fats, and nutrient-dense sides, setting the stage for sustainable health and vitality.

# Chapter 1: Overview of the Primal diet, and its core principles.

The Primal Diet is a nutritional approach inspired by the eating habits of early humans, focusing on whole, unprocessed foods.

**Its core principles include:**
- ❖ High Protein and Healthy Fats: Emphasizing lean meats (grass-fed, wild-caught), fish, eggs, and healthy fats from sources like avocados and nuts while minimizing carbohydrates.
- ❖ Abundant Vegetables: Encouraging a wide variety of non-starchy vegetables to ensure nutrient diversity.
- ❖ Avoidance of Processed Foods: Excluding grains, sugars, and artificial additives that are detrimental to health.

## The benefits of meat-based nutrition and how it differs from other diets.

- ❖ Meat-based nutrition offers numerous benefits that distinguish it from other dietary approaches. Key advantages include:
- ❖ Nutrient Density: Meat is rich in essential nutrients like protein, iron, zinc, and vitamin B12, which are crucial for muscle growth, brain health, and overall vitality. These nutrients are often more bioavailable in meat than in plant sources.
- ❖ Health Benefits: Studies indicate that meat consumption can lead to improved energy levels, mental clarity, and weight management. For instance, a 2021 study found that individuals on a carnivore diet reported significant health improvements, including weight loss and better metabolic markers.
- ❖ Muscle Maintenance: High-quality animal proteins support muscle growth and maintenance, particularly important as people age. This helps prevent conditions like sarcopenia (muscle wasting) and supports overall strength.

❖ Balanced Blood Sugar: Unlike many carbohydrate-rich diets, meat has a low glycemic load, which helps maintain stable blood sugar levels and reduces the risk of insulin resistance.

## common misconceptions about meat in a balanced way, supported by research:

Common misconceptions about meat consumption often lead to confusion regarding its health implications. Here are some balanced insights supported by research:

❖ Meat and Heart Disease: Critics often claim that meat, especially red and processed varieties, significantly increases the risk of cardiovascular diseases. While some studies indicate a correlation, particularly with processed meats, the evidence is nuanced. For instance, a systematic review found weak associations between unprocessed red meat and major health outcomes like ischemic heart disease and diabetes, suggesting that factors like body mass index (BMI) play a significant role in these risks.

❖ Cancer Risks: The World Health Organization has linked processed meat to colorectal cancer; however, the association with unprocessed red meat is less clear. Some meta-analyses show minimal risk increase, indicating that when consumed as part of a balanced diet, unprocessed red meat may not pose significant cancer risks.

❖ Nutritional Benefits: Meat is a rich source of bioavailable nutrients essential for health, including high-quality protein, iron, and vitamin B12. These nutrients are vital for muscle maintenance and overall vitality, particularly in populations at risk for deficiencies.

❖ Type 2 Diabetes: While studies suggest higher red meat consumption correlates with increased diabetes risk, replacing red meat with plant-based proteins has shown to lower this risk significantly. This highlights the importance of dietary balance rather than outright elimination of meat.

**Concept of "Primal Plate" and set the tone for a guide that values high-quality meat, healthy fats, and nutrient-rich sides.**

The concept of the "Primal Plate" embodies a holistic approach to nutrition, emphasizing high-quality meats, healthy fats, and nutrient-dense vegetables. This lifestyle is rooted in the belief that our bodies thrive on the foods our ancestors consumed, promoting optimal health through whole, unprocessed foods.

The Primal Plate encourages:

- ❖ High-Quality Meat: Prioritizing grass-fed, pasture-raised, and wild-caught options to ensure nutrient density and ethical sourcing.
- ❖ Healthy Fats: Including sources like avocados, nuts, and oils (e.g., olive and coconut) for energy and essential fatty acids.
- ❖ Nutrient-Rich Sides: Incorporating a variety of colorful vegetables to provide vitamins, minerals, and fiber.

Setting the tone for this guide, the Primal Plate advocates for a balanced diet that not only supports physical health but also fosters a sustainable lifestyle. By focusing on nutrient-dense foods and avoiding processed items, readers are empowered to make informed choices that enhance their overall well-being.

# Chapter 2: Health Benefits of a Meat-First Diet.

A meat-based diet offers several primary health benefits, which set it apart from other dietary approaches:

- **Weight Loss:** High-protein diets, particularly those rich in meat, can enhance satiety, leading to reduced calorie intake. Studies show that participants on a meat-centric diet often experience significant weight loss due to increased protein consumption and lower carbohydrate intake, which promotes fat burning and reduces water retention from glycogen stores.
- **Increased Mental Clarity:** Many individuals report improved cognitive function and mental clarity when consuming a meat-first diet. This is attributed to the bioavailable nutrients found in meat, such as omega-3 fatty acids and B vitamins, which support brain health and mood stabilization.
- **Reduced Inflammation:** Meat contains anti-inflammatory properties and lacks the glycemic load associated with many carbohydrate-rich foods. By replacing inflammatory grains and sugars with nutrient-dense meats, individuals may experience lower levels of systemic inflammation, contributing to overall health improvements.
- **Higher Energy Levels:** The nutrient density of meat provides sustained energy. Dieters often report increased energy levels and enhanced physical performance due to the high-quality protein and fats that fuel the body effectively.

## A meat-based diet supports wellness across various areas, including physical health and mood stability, through several mechanisms:

- **Physical Health:** Meat is a rich source of essential nutrients such as protein, iron, and B vitamins, which are vital for muscle maintenance, energy production, and overall bodily functions. These nutrients help improve metabolic efficiency and support immune function, contributing to better physical health outcomes.
- **Mood Stability:** Research indicates that meat consumption is associated with lower rates of depression and anxiety compared to vegetarian diets. A

systematic review found that individuals who consume meat generally report better psychological health, suggesting that the nutrients in meat may play a role in enhancing mood stability. Specifically, nutrients like vitamin B12 and omega-3 fatty acids found in animal products are linked to improved mental health outcomes and reduced depressive symptoms.

- **Cognitive Function:** A diet rich in high-quality proteins from meat can enhance cognitive function and mental clarity. Studies show that adequate protein intake is crucial for neurotransmitter synthesis, which affects mood and cognitive processes. This suggests that a meat-first diet may contribute to better focus and mental performance.
- **Reduced Inflammation:** Meat contains anti-inflammatory properties that can help lower systemic inflammation, which is often linked to mood disorders. By minimizing inflammatory markers in the body, a meat-based diet may promote a more stable emotional state.

## Scientific studies and expert insights supporting the health benefits of a meat-based diet:

- **Weight Loss:** A 2021 study by Harvard researchers found that participants on a carnivore diet experienced significant weight loss, with 93% reporting improvements in obesity and excess weight. This diet was associated with high satisfaction and few adverse effects, highlighting its effectiveness for weight management.
- **Increased Mental Clarity:** Research indicates that meat consumption is linked to better mood and mental health. A comprehensive analysis revealed that individuals who eat meat have lower rates of depression and anxiety compared to vegetarians and vegans, suggesting that nutrients like vitamin B12 and omega-3 fatty acids found in meat may enhance cognitive function.
- **Reduced Inflammation:** Many advocates of the carnivore diet report reductions in inflammation-related symptoms. This aligns with findings that a diet low in carbohydrates can lower systemic inflammation, which is beneficial for overall health.
- **Higher Energy Levels:** Participants in the aforementioned Harvard study reported increased energy levels after adopting a carnivore diet. The nutrient

density of meat provides sustained energy, supporting physical performance and daily activities.

density of meat provides sustained energy, supporting physical performance and daily activities.

# Chapter 3: Science and Nutrition – Understanding Meat-Based Diets

Science-based overview of how the body responds positively to a meat-first diet.

A meat-first diet, or Primal Diet, positively influences the body through various mechanisms that enhance overall health and well-being:

- **Nutrient Density:** Meat is a rich source of essential nutrients, including high-quality protein, iron, zinc, and B vitamins. These nutrients are crucial for muscle repair, energy production, and cognitive function. Studies show that meat provides bioavailable forms of these nutrients that are often lacking in plant-based diets.
- **Metabolic Benefits:** Research indicates that diets high in protein, particularly from meat sources, can improve metabolic efficiency. A study highlighted that participants on high-meat diets exhibited better cardiovascular health and weight loss outcomes compared to those on lower-meat diets. This suggests that meat consumption can support weight management and metabolic health.
- **Reduced Inflammation:** Meat contains anti-inflammatory properties that can help lower systemic inflammation. A meta-analysis found no significant link between saturated fat from meat and increased cardiovascular disease risk, challenging the notion that meat is inherently harmful. This reduction in inflammation may contribute to improved overall health.
- **Cognitive Function:** Nutrients found in meat, such as omega-3 fatty acids and B vitamins, are linked to enhanced cognitive function. Studies suggest that adequate intake of these nutrients supports brain health and mood stabilization

## The roles of protein, healthy fats, and micronutrients found in animal products for cellular repair, brain health, and metabolic efficiency.

Animal products play a crucial role in supporting cellular repair, brain health, and metabolic efficiency through their rich content of protein, healthy fats, and micronutrients:

Protein

- **Cellular Repair and Growth:** Protein is essential for the synthesis of new cells and the repair of damaged tissues. Amino acids, the building blocks of proteins, play critical roles in various bodily functions, including hormone production and immune response. For instance, leucine, an essential amino acid found abundantly in meat, is particularly effective at stimulating muscle protein synthesis, which is vital for recovery after exercise and injury .
- **Muscle Maintenance:** A diet rich in animal protein helps preserve lean muscle mass, especially important as we age. Research shows that higher protein intake can counteract sarcopenia (age-related muscle loss) by promoting muscle strength and function. This is crucial not only for physical performance but also for maintaining metabolic rate since muscle tissue burns more calories at rest than fat tissue .

## Healthy Fats

- **Brain Health:** Healthy fats from animal sources, particularly omega-3 fatty acids (EPA and DHA), are integral to brain structure and function. These fats contribute to the formation of cell membranes and are involved in neurotransmitter signaling. Studies have shown that adequate intake of omega-3s is associated with reduced risk of cognitive decline and improved mood stability .
- **Hormonal Balance:** Fats are essential for hormone production, including sex hormones like testosterone and estrogen. Healthy fats also support the absorption of fat-soluble vitamins (A, D, E, K), which are crucial for various physiological processes. For example, vitamin D plays a significant role in calcium metabolism and immune function .
- **Energy Production:** Fats provide a concentrated source of energy (9 calories per gram), which is particularly beneficial during prolonged physical activity or low-carbohydrate diets. The body can efficiently utilize fats for energy through a process called ketosis, where fat stores are converted into ketones that serve as an alternative fuel source .

# Micronutrients

- ❖ Essential Vitamins: Animal products are rich in several vitamins that are less abundant in plant foods. For example:
  - ➢ **Vitamin B12:** Essential for neurological function and DNA synthesis; deficiency can lead to anemia and neurological disorders .
  - ➢ **Vitamin A:** Critical for vision, immune function, and skin health; animal sources (like liver) provide retinol, the active form of vitamin A that is more readily absorbed than carotenoids from plants.
- ❖ **Minerals:**
  - ➢ **Iron:** Heme iron from meat is more bioavailable than non-heme iron from plant sources. This is crucial for preventing iron-deficiency anemia, which can impair oxygen transport and energy levels .
  - ➢ **Zinc:** Important for immune function, wound healing, and DNA synthesis; meat is one of the best dietary sources of zinc .
  - ➢ **Selenium:** Found in high amounts in meats like beef and poultry, selenium acts as an antioxidant that protects cells from oxidative stress.

# Scientific Insights on Meat-Based Diets

A meat-based diet offers numerous health benefits supported by scientific research. Below are key points and findings that illustrate how the body responds positively to a meat-first approach.

## Protein and Cellular Repair

- High Biological Value: Animal proteins are complete, containing all essential amino acids necessary for tissue repair and growth. A study published in The American Journal of Clinical Nutrition emphasizes that high-protein diets can enhance muscle synthesis, vital for recovery and overall health.

## Healthy Fats and Brain Health

- Omega-3 Fatty Acids: Found in fatty fish and grass-fed meats, omega-3s are crucial for cognitive function. Research indicates that adequate intake of omega-3s is associated with reduced risk of cognitive decline and improved mood stability.

## Micronutrients for Metabolic Efficiency

- Iron Bioavailability: Heme iron from meat is more easily absorbed than non-heme iron from plant sources. This is particularly important for preventing iron-deficiency anemia, which can impair energy levels and cognitive function. A systematic review highlighted that meat consumption is positively associated with better iron status in children, enhancing growth and cognitive outcomes.

## Sidebar: Interesting Facts

- Protein Utilization: Studies show that dietary protein from animal sources is utilized more efficiently by the body compared to plant proteins, making it a superior choice for muscle maintenance and repair.
- Nutrient Density: A 100g serving of lean beef provides approximately 26g of protein, 2.6mg of iron, and significant amounts of zinc and B vitamins, demonstrating its nutrient density compared to many plant-based foods.

## Diagram of Nutrient Roles in a Meat-Based Diet

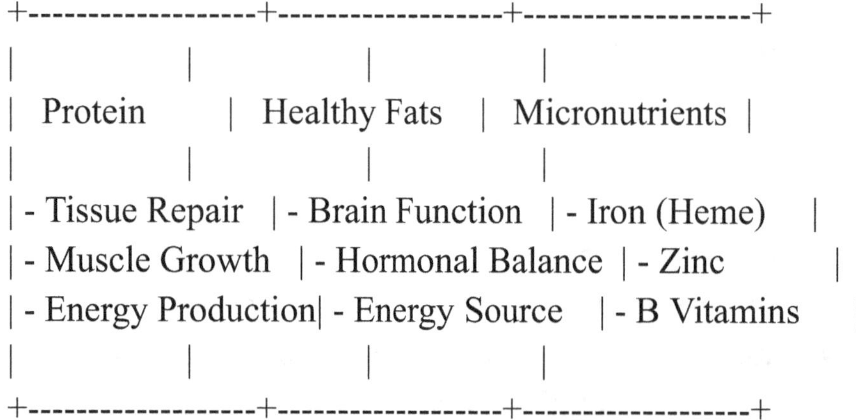

```
+-------------------+-------------------+-------------------+
|                   |                   |                   |
|  Protein          |  Healthy Fats     |  Micronutrients   |
|                   |                   |                   |
| - Tissue Repair   | - Brain Function  | - Iron (Heme)     |
| - Muscle Growth   | - Hormonal Balance| - Zinc            |
| - Energy Production| - Energy Source  | - B Vitamins      |
|                   |                   |                   |
+-------------------+-------------------+-------------------+
```

This diagram illustrates the essential roles of protein, healthy fats, and micronutrients found in animal products, emphasizing their contributions to cellular repair, brain health, and metabolic efficiency.

# Chapter 4: Crafting a Balanced Meat-First Diet Plan

To create a balanced meat-first diet, it's essential to incorporate a variety of meats—each offering unique nutrients that contribute to overall health. Here's how to balance different types of meats for diverse nutrient intake while ensuring your meals are satisfying and nutritious.

## Types of Meats and Their Nutritional Benefits

- ❖ **Red Meat (Beef, Lamb, Pork)**
  - ➤ Nutrients: High in iron, zinc, and B vitamins (especially B12).
  - ➤ Benefits: Red meat is an excellent source of heme iron, which is more readily absorbed by the body than non-heme iron from plant sources. It supports energy levels and helps prevent anemia. A study found that red meat consumption is associated with improved muscle mass and strength due to its high protein content .
  - ➤ Serving Suggestions: Opt for lean cuts like sirloin or tenderloin to reduce saturated fat intake. Incorporate red meat into stews, stir-fries, or grilled dishes.

- ❖ **Poultry (Chicken, Turkey)**
  - ➤ Nutrients: Lean source of protein, niacin, and selenium.
  - ➤ Benefits: Poultry is lower in saturated fat compared to red meat, making it heart-healthy. It provides essential amino acids for muscle maintenance and contains nutrients that support immune function. Epidemiological studies suggest that regular poultry consumption is linked to a reduced risk of obesity and cardiovascular diseases .
  - ➤ Serving Suggestions: Use skinless chicken breasts or thighs in salads, soups, or casseroles. Roast whole chickens for versatile meal prep options.

- ❖ **Fish (Salmon, Mackerel, Sardines)**
  - ➤ Nutrients: Rich in omega-3 fatty acids, vitamin D, and iodine.
  - ➤ Benefits: Omega-3s are crucial for brain health and reducing inflammation. Regular fish consumption has been shown to improve heart health and cognitive function. The American Heart Association

recommends eating fish at least twice a week for its numerous health benefits .

- ➤ Serving Suggestions: Grill or bake fish with herbs and lemon for added flavor. Incorporate canned fish like sardines into salads or pasta dishes for convenience.
- ❖ **Organ Meats (Liver, Kidney)**
    - ➤ Nutrients: Extremely nutrient-dense; high in vitamin A, B vitamins (especially B12), iron, and copper.
    - ➤ Benefits: Organ meats provide some of the highest concentrations of essential nutrients per serving. Liver is particularly beneficial for its vitamin A content, which supports vision and immune function. Including organ meats can enhance overall nutrient intake without requiring large portion sizes .
    - ➤ Serving Suggestions: Incorporate liver into pâtés or sauté it with onions for a flavorful dish. Use kidney in stews or pies for added richness.

## Balancing Your Meat Intake

- ❖ Portion Control: Aim for moderate portions of each type of meat to prevent excessive calorie intake while ensuring a variety of nutrients:
    - ➤ Red Meat: Limit to about 70g cooked weight per day to reduce health risks associated with high consumption .
    - ➤ Poultry: Include skinless options; about 80g cooked weight is recommended.
    - ➤ Fish: Aim for at least two servings per week (approximately 100g per serving).
- ❖ Diverse Protein Sources: While focusing on meat, consider integrating other protein sources such as eggs, legumes (lentils, chickpeas), nuts (almonds, walnuts), and seeds (chia seeds) into your meals. This diversification ensures a broader range of nutrients while maintaining a meat-centric diet.

## Complementing with Nutrient-Rich Foods

To enhance the nutritional value of your meals:

❖ **Pairing with Vegetables:** Incorporate a variety of colorful vegetables to increase fiber intake and provide antioxidants. Aim for at least half your plate to be filled with vegetables at each meal.
  ➢ Examples: Roasted Brussels sprouts with beef; sautéed spinach with chicken; or grilled zucchini with salmon.
❖ **Healthy Carbohydrate Sources:** Consider adding whole grains or legumes as side dishes to provide complex carbohydrates and additional protein.
  ➢ Examples: Quinoa salad with grilled chicken; brown rice served with stir-fried vegetables and beef; or lentil soup paired with roasted chicken.
❖ **Healthy Cooking Methods:** Use cooking methods that preserve nutrients while minimizing added fats:
  ➢ Grilling, baking, steaming, or slow cooking can enhance flavors without the need for excessive oils or fats.

## Meal Planning Tips

❖ Weekly Meal Prep:
  ➢ Dedicate time each week to plan meals around your chosen meats. Prepare large batches of proteins that can be used in various dishes throughout the week.
  ➢ For example, roast a whole chicken on Sunday that can be used in salads, sandwiches, or soups during the week.
❖ Shopping List Creation:
  ➢ Create a shopping list that includes diverse types of meats along with vegetables and healthy fats (like olive oil or avocado). This ensures you have all the ingredients needed for balanced meals.
❖ Experimenting with Recipes:
  ➢ Explore different cuisines that highlight various meats—such as Mediterranean (lamb), Asian (chicken stir-fry), or Scandinavian (fish dishes)—to keep meals exciting.

## Sidebar: Interesting Facts

- **Iron Absorption Boost:** Consuming vitamin C-rich foods (like bell peppers or citrus fruits) alongside meat can significantly enhance the absorption of nonheme iron from plant sources.
- **Bioavailability:** The heme iron found in red meat has an absorption rate of approximately 23%, compared to only 2-8% for non-heme iron from plant sources .

## Suggest portions, meal timing, and complementary vegetables or sides to create a well-rounded plate.

Creating a balanced meat-first diet involves thoughtful portioning, meal timing, and pairing meats with complementary vegetables and sides. This approach ensures you receive a diverse range of nutrients while enjoying satisfying meals. Suggested Portions for Different Meats:

- ❖ Red Meat (Beef, Lamb, Pork)
    - ➢ Recommended Portion: 70–100g cooked (about the size of a deck of cards).
    - ➢ Weekly Limit: Aim for a maximum of 500g per week to reduce health risks associated with high consumption .
    - ➢ Serving Suggestions: Use lean cuts like sirloin or tenderloin, and incorporate into stews or grilled dishes.
- ❖ Poultry (Chicken, Turkey)
    - ➢ Recommended Portion: 80–120g cooked (about the size of a palm).
    - ➢ Weekly Limit: 2–3 servings per week.
    - ➢ Serving Suggestions: Skinless chicken breasts can be roasted or grilled and added to salads or stir-fries.
- ❖ Fish (Salmon, Mackerel, Sardines)
    - ➢ Recommended Portion: 100g cooked (approximately the size of a small filet).
    - ➢ Weekly Limit: At least two servings per week.
    - ➢ Serving Suggestions: Grill or bake fish with herbs and lemon; consider canned options for quick meals.
- ❖ Organ Meats (Liver, Kidney)

> ➤ Recommended Portion: 50–100g cooked (about the size of a small palm).
> ➤ Weekly Limit: Once per week is sufficient.
> ➤ Serving Suggestions: Incorporate liver into pâtés or sauté it with onions for added flavor.

## Meal Timing Recommendations

- ❖ **Breakfast:** Aim to include a source of protein within two hours of waking to kickstart metabolism. Consider options like scrambled eggs with spinach or Greek yogurt with nuts.
- ❖ **Lunch:** Include a balanced portion of meat (e.g., grilled chicken salad) along with plenty of vegetables to maintain energy levels throughout the afternoon.
- ❖ **Dinner:** Focus on a larger protein portion (e.g., roasted beef with steamed broccoli) accompanied by healthy fats (olive oil dressing) and fiber-rich vegetables.
- ❖ **Snacks:** Incorporate protein-rich snacks such as hard-boiled eggs, jerky, or a handful of nuts to sustain energy levels between meals.

## Complementary Vegetables and Sides

To enhance the nutritional value of your meals, pair meats with a variety of vegetables and whole grains:

- ❖ **Leafy Greens:** Spinach, kale, and Swiss chard are rich in vitamins A, C, and K. They can be used in salads or sautéed as sides.
- ❖ **Cruciferous Vegetables:** Broccoli, cauliflower, and Brussels sprouts provide fiber and antioxidants. Roast them alongside meats for added flavor.
- ❖ **Colorful Vegetables:** Bell peppers, carrots, and beets offer a range of nutrients. Use them in stir-fries or as raw snacks with dips.
- ❖ Whole Grains: Quinoa, brown rice, or farro can complement meat dishes while providing complex carbohydrates for sustained energy.
- ❖ **Legumes:** Lentils and chickpeas add protein and fiber; they can be included in salads or served as side dishes.

**Meal Example**

**Here's an example of a well-rounded meat-first meal:**
- ❖ Grilled Chicken Breast (100g) served over a bed of mixed greens (spinach, arugula) topped with cherry tomatoes and avocado slices.
- ❖ Roasted Brussels Sprouts drizzled with olive oil.
- ❖ A side of quinoa salad mixed with diced cucumbers and parsley.

## Sidebar: Interesting Facts

- **Iron Absorption Boost:** Consuming vitamin C-rich foods (like bell peppers or citrus fruits) alongside meat can significantly enhance the absorption of nonheme iron from plant sources.
- **Protein Timing:** Research indicates that distributing protein intake evenly across meals—aiming for about 25–30g at each meal—can maximize muscle protein synthesis throughout the day .

## Tips on combining flavors, maximizing nutrient density, and adjusting meal plans based on dietary needs.

Creating delicious and nutritious meals in a meat-first diet involves thoughtful combinations of flavors, maximizing nutrient density, and adjusting meal plans based on individual dietary needs. Here are some practical tips to help you achieve this:

**Combining Flavors**
- ❖ **Contrast and Complement:**
  - ➢ Pair rich, savory meats with bright, acidic elements to enhance flavor. For example, grilled chicken can be complemented with a citrus vinaigrette or a squeeze of lemon to balance richness.
  - ➢ Use sweet elements to contrast savory dishes. For instance, adding a touch of honey or maple syrup to a marinade for pork can create a delightful glaze.
- ❖ **Herbs and Spices:**
  - ➢ Fresh herbs like basil, cilantro, or parsley can elevate the flavor profile of meat dishes. For example, marinating steak with rosemary and garlic adds depth.

➢ Experiment with spices such as cumin or paprika to add warmth and complexity. A spice blend can transform simple grilled meats into flavorful dishes.

❖ **Flavor Pairings:**
➢ Classic combinations like olive oil, feta cheese, and fresh lemon juice create a Mediterranean flair that enhances salads or roasted meats .
➢ Consider unique pairings like prosciutto wrapped around melon or figs; the sweetness of the fruit complements the saltiness of the meat .

**Maximizing Nutrient Density**

❖ **Incorporate Variety:**
➢ Include different types of meats (red meat, poultry, fish, organ meats) in your diet to ensure a broad spectrum of nutrients. Each type offers unique vitamins and minerals essential for health.
➢ Add nutrient-dense vegetables like leafy greens (spinach, kale), cruciferous veggies (broccoli, cauliflower), and colorful peppers to meals for added fiber, vitamins, and antioxidants.

❖ **Healthy Fats:**
➢ Use healthy fats such as olive oil or avocado oil when cooking or dressing salads to enhance nutrient absorption (especially fat-soluble vitamins A, D, E, and K).
➢ Incorporate sources of omega-3 fatty acids from fish like salmon or mackerel for heart health and anti-inflammatory benefits .

❖ **Whole Grains and Legumes:**
➢ When appropriate, include whole grains (quinoa, brown rice) or legumes (lentils, chickpeas) as side dishes to provide complex carbohydrates and additional protein.
➢ Adjusting Meal Plans Based on Dietary Needs

❖ Personalization:
➢ Consider individual dietary requirements such as food allergies, intolerances (e.g., gluten), or specific health conditions (e.g., diabetes). Adjust portion sizes and food choices accordingly.
➢ For those needing lower fat intake, opt for lean cuts of meat (like skinless chicken breast) and limit fatty cuts or processed meats.

❖ **Meal Timing:**

> ➤ Plan meals around activity levels; for example, consume higher protein meals post-workout to support muscle recovery.
> ➤ Distribute protein intake evenly across meals to maximize muscle protein synthesis throughout the day .

❖ **Batch Cooking:**
> ➤ Prepare larger quantities of proteins (like roasted chicken or beef stew) that can be portioned out for quick meals during busy days.
> ➤ Freeze portions for later use; this ensures you have healthy options readily available without the need for daily cooking.

❖ **Seasonal Adjustments:**
> ➤ Adapt meal plans based on seasonal availability of produce; this not only enhances flavor but also ensures freshness and nutrient density.
> ➤ Experiment with different cooking methods based on the season—grilling in summer versus slow-cooking in winter can bring variety to your meals.

# Chapter 5: Essential Kitchen Tools and Techniques for Meat Preparation.

## Essential Kitchen Tools for Meat Preparation

### 1. Meat Thermometer

A meat thermometer is an indispensable tool for any cook. It ensures that meat reaches the appropriate internal temperature, which is crucial for both safety and flavor. There are several types of meat thermometers:

- Instant-Read Thermometers: Provide quick readings, ideal for checking doneness.
- Probe Thermometers: Can be left in the meat while it cooks, allowing you to monitor the temperature without opening the oven or grill.

### 2. Cast Iron Pan

Cast iron pans are renowned for their heat retention and even cooking. They are perfect for:

- Searing: Achieving a beautiful crust on steaks and chops.
- Oven-to-Table Cooking: Transitioning from stovetop to oven seamlessly.
- Versatility: Great for frying, baking, and even slow cooking.

### 3. Slow Cooker

Slow cookers are fantastic for preparing tender, flavorful meals with minimal effort. They excel in:

- Braising: Perfect for tougher cuts of meat that benefit from long cooking times.
- Convenience: Set it in the morning and return to a delicious meal.
- Flavor Development: Allows flavors to meld over time, enhancing the overall taste.

### 4. Dutch Oven

A Dutch oven is a heavy-duty pot that can be used on the stovetop or in the oven. Its benefits include:

- Even Heat Distribution: Ensures consistent cooking results.
- Versatility: Suitable for braising, stewing, roasting, and baking.
- Durability: Often made from cast iron, it can last a lifetime with proper care.

## 5. Chef's Knife

A high-quality chef's knife is essential for meat preparation. It allows for:
- Precision Cutting: For slicing, dicing, and trimming meat efficiently.
- Versatility: Useful for a variety of tasks beyond just meat preparation.

## 6. Cutting Board

A sturdy cutting board provides a safe surface for cutting and preparing meat. Consider:
- Material: Wood or plastic boards are common; choose one that is easy to clean and maintain.
- Size: Ensure it's large enough to handle bigger cuts of meat without crowding.

## 7. Meat Mallet or Tenderizer

A meat mallet is useful for tenderizing tougher cuts of meat before cooking. It helps:
- Break Down Fibers: Making meat more tender and easier to chew.
- Even Cooking: Ensures uniform thickness for even cooking.

## 8. Marinade Injector

For those who love flavor-packed meats, a marinade injector allows you to infuse marinades directly into the meat, ensuring maximum flavor throughout.

## 9. Food Processor

A food processor can be invaluable when preparing ground meats or making marinades and sauces quickly and efficiently.

# Techniques for Effective Meat Preparation

### 1. Proper Seasoning

Seasoning your meat with salt and spices before cooking enhances its natural flavors. Consider marinating or dry brining to infuse flavor deeply.

### 2. Resting Meat

Allow cooked meat to rest before slicing. This helps redistribute juices, resulting in a juicier final product.

### 3. Searing Techniques

Searing meat at high temperatures creates a flavorful crust through the Maillard reaction, adding depth to your dishes.

### 4. Basting

Basting meats during cooking (especially in the oven) keeps them moist and adds flavor from any fats or seasonings used.

### 5. Cutting Against the Grain

When slicing cooked meats, always cut against the grain to ensure tenderness in each bite.

## Cooking techniques like searing, roasting, and smoking that enhance the flavor and texture of different cuts.

### 1. Searing

Searing is a foundational technique that locks in moisture and adds rich flavor through browning. Here's how to make the most of it:

**Technique:**

- **Preheat the Pan:** Use a heavy skillet or cast iron pan and heat it until it's very hot.
- **Pat Dry:** Ensure the meat is dry before seasoning to promote browning.

- **Use Oil with High Smoke Point:** Oils like canola, grapeseed, or avocado oil work best.
- **Do Not Crowd the Pan:** Sear in batches if necessary to maintain high heat.

**Best Cuts for Searing:**
- Steaks: Ribeye, sirloin, and filet mignon benefit greatly from searing.
- Pork Chops: Thick-cut chops develop a beautiful crust.
- Chicken Breasts: Searing skin-on chicken helps render fat and crisp the skin.

## 2. Roasting

Enhancing the flavor and texture of meat involves mastering various cooking techniques. Here are some key methods:

**Technique:**
- Season Generously: Use salt, pepper, and herbs to season your meat before roasting.
- Use a Rack: Elevate the meat on a rack in the roasting pan to allow air circulation and even cooking.
- Baste Occasionally: Baste with pan juices or broth to keep the meat moist.

**Best Cuts for Roasting:**
- Whole Chicken or Turkey: Roasting brings out natural flavors and creates crispy skin.
- Beef Roasts: Cuts like prime rib or tenderloin are perfect for roasting.
- Pork Loin: A flavorful cut that benefits from slow roasting.

## 3. Smoking

Smoking adds depth and complexity to meats through low and slow cooking with wood smoke.

**Technique:**
- Choose Your Wood Wisely: Different woods impart different flavors; hickory, mesquite, applewood, and cherry are popular choices.

- Maintain Low Temperatures: Aim for 225°F to 250°F for hot smoking; cold smoking should be below 90°F.
- Use a Water Pan: Placing a water pan in the smoker helps maintain moisture.

**Best Cuts for Smoking:**

- Brisket: A classic choice that becomes tender and flavorful when smoked for hours.
- Pork Ribs: Smoking enhances their natural sweetness while creating a tender texture.
- Salmon: Cold smoking adds a delicate flavor without cooking the fish through.

## 4. Braising

Braising combines both dry and wet cooking methods, making it ideal for tougher cuts of meat.

**Technique:**

- Sear First: Begin by searing the meat to develop flavor.
- Add Liquid: Use broth, wine, or even beer to create steam and moisture during cooking.
- Low and Slow Cooking: Cover tightly and cook at low temperatures (around 300°F) for several hours until tender.

**Best Cuts for Braising:**

- Chuck Roast: Perfect for pot roast; becomes incredibly tender when braised.
- Short Ribs: Rich in flavor; braising breaks down connective tissue.
- Pork Shoulder: Ideal for pulled pork; becomes melt-in-your-mouth tender.

5. Grilling

Grilling is another fantastic method that imparts a smoky flavor while achieving a charred exterior.

**Technique:**

- Preheat the Grill: Ensure your grill is hot before adding meat.

- Oil the Grates: Prevent sticking by oiling the grill grates before placing meat on them.
- Direct vs. Indirect Heat: Use direct heat for quick-cooking cuts (like steaks) and indirect heat for larger cuts (like whole chickens).

**Best Cuts for Grilling:**
- Steaks: Ribeye, flank, and T-bone are great choices.
- Chicken Thighs or Drumsticks: Skin-on pieces retain moisture while grilling.
- Vegetables and Fruit: Enhance your meal by grilling seasonal vegetables or fruits like peaches.

# Practical advice on marinating, seasoning, and achieving restaurant-quality results at home.

## Advanced Marinating Techniques
- Layering Flavors: Consider using multiple layers of flavor in your marinade. Start with a base of acid (like yogurt or buttermilk for chicken), then add herbs, spices, and aromatics (like garlic or ginger) to build complexity.
- Incorporate Sweetness: Adding a sweet element (like honey, brown sugar, or fruit juice) can balance acidity and enhance caramelization during cooking. This is particularly effective for grilling.
- Use a Vacuum Sealer: For maximum flavor penetration, use a vacuum sealer to marinate meat. The vacuum environment helps the marinade infuse deeper into the meat fibers.
- Experiment with Different Acids: Different acidic ingredients can impart unique flavors. Try using citrus juices (lemon, lime, orange), vinegars (balsamic, apple cider), or even wine to vary the taste of your dishes.

## Enhanced Seasoning Techniques
- Salt Types: Experiment with different types of salt. Coarse sea salt or kosher salt is great for seasoning meat before cooking, while fine sea salt can be used for finishing touches.

- Brining: For lean meats like chicken breasts or pork chops, consider bringing them in a saltwater solution (with optional sugar and spices) for several hours before cooking. This helps retain moisture and enhances flavor.
- Finishing Salts: Use finishing salts (like fleur de sel or smoked salt) just before serving to add a burst of flavor and texture. These salts can elevate the dish's presentation and taste.

**Achieving Restaurant-Quality Cooking Techniques**

**1. Sous Vide Cooking**
- Precision Cooking: Sous vide involves vacuum-sealing food in a bag and cooking it to a precise temperature in a water bath. This method ensures perfect doneness and retains moisture.
- Finishing Touches: After sous vide cooking, quickly sear the meat in a hot pan for that desirable crust.

**2. Basting**
- Flavor Infusion: Basting meats with their own juices or a flavored butter during cooking adds moisture and enhances flavor. For example, baste chicken with herb-infused butter while roasting.

**3. Deglazing**
- Flavor Development: After searing meat, use wine or broth to deglaze the pan by scraping up the browned bits stuck to the bottom. This creates a flavorful base for sauces that can accompany your dish.

**4. Resting and Slicing**
- Proper Resting: Allow meats to rest covered loosely with foil after cooking; this helps retain juices. The general rule is to rest larger cuts for 10-15 minutes and smaller cuts for 5-10 minutes.
- Slicing Technique: Always slice against the grain for tenderness. For larger cuts like brisket or pork shoulder, let them cool slightly before slicing to help maintain their structure.

## Plating and Presentation

- Visual Appeal: Take time to plate your dish beautifully. Use contrasting colors (like vibrant vegetables alongside golden-brown meat) and consider height in plating to create an appealing presentation.
- Garnishes: Fresh herbs, microgreens, or edible flowers can add color and freshness to your plate. A drizzle of high-quality olive oil or balsamic reduction can also enhance visual appeal.

## Creating Sauces and Accompaniments

- Homemade Sauces: Elevate your dish with homemade sauces like chimichurri, salsa verde, or classic pan sauces made from drippings.
- Pairing Sides Thoughtfully: Consider complementary flavors when choosing sides; roasted vegetables with herbs go well with grilled meats, while creamy polenta pairs nicely with braised dishes.

# Chapter 6: Sourcing Quality Meat and Ingredients

Choosing high-quality, ethically sourced meats is critical to both health and sustainability. Here's how to choose the best options:

## 1. Understanding Meat Labels.

**Grass-Fed:** Cattle were grown on pasture and fed grass instead of grain. This frequently leads to leaner meat with more omega-3 fatty acids.

**Pasture-Raised:** Animals are free to graze outside, which improves their quality of life and the flavor of the meat.

Wild-caught refers to fish and shellfish caught in their native environments. Wild-caught fish typically have superior nutritional profiles than farmed versions.

## 2. Sourcing Quality Meat

**Local farms:** Look for local farms that use sustainable farming practices. Visiting farmers' markets can provide information on how animals are raised.

**Certified Labels:** Look for certificates such as Certified Humane, Animal Welfare Approved, or USDA Organic, which suggest higher welfare standards.

**Butcher Shops:** Develop ties with local butchers who may share information on sourcing and handling techniques.

## 3. Choosing seafood.

**Sustainable Options:** Use tools such as the Monterey Bay Seafood Watch app to find sustainably sourced seafood. When feasible, choose wild-caught choices because they contain fewer contaminants.

Avoid overfished species. Be wary of species that are overfished or caught via harmful methods. Choose species that are abundant and caught responsibly.

## 4. Nutritional Considerations.

Healthy fats: Grass-fed and pasture-raised meats often have healthier fats than conventionally grown meats, which contributes to improved heart health.

Ethically sourced meats frequently have deeper flavors due to their diets and living conditions, which improves the whole culinary experience.

# 5. Cooking with high-quality ingredients.

**Preparation Techniques:** High-quality meats frequently require simpler cooking methods (such as grilling or roasting) to bring out their natural flavors.

**Seasoning:** Use minimal seasoning to let the natural flavors of sustainably sourced meats shine through.

# 6. Recognize Quality Indicators

**When shopping for beef, seek for key markers of quality:**
**Visual Inspection**
**Color:** Fresh beef should be bright red, while lamb should be a rich pink. Pork is normally light pink, whereas poultry should be pale in color. Avoid meat that seems dull or has an odd color.

Look for intramuscular fat (marbling) in cuts such as steak. Good marbling suggests softness and taste.

**Texture:** The meat should be firm and slightly juicy, but not sticky or slimy.
Smell
Fresh meat should smell clean and mild. A strong or sour odor indicates that the meat is not fresh.

# 7. Ethical Sourcing Practices.

Understanding the practices behind meat production might help you make informed decisions.
Animal Welfare Standards

**Free range versus cage-free:** Free-range animals have access to the outdoors, whereas cage-free birds are not kept in cages but may still have limited area. Look for certifications indicating greater welfare requirements.

**Grass-fed versus grain-finished:** While grass-fed calves are healthier and produce leaner meat, some farmers finish their cattle on grain for a short time to increase marbling. Understanding the animal's full lifecycle might help you make a decision depending on your preferences.
Environmental Impact

**Sustainable farming practices:** Look for farms that use rotational grazing, which improves soil health while reducing environmental effect.

**Reduced Antibiotic Use:** Choose meat from producers who use fewer antibiotics, as this contributes to antibiotic resistance in humans.

## 8. Shopping Tips

**Know your sources:** Look into local farms, co-ops, and butcher shops that value ethical sourcing. Many farms provide subscription services that provide regular deliveries of high-quality meats.

**Ask questions:** Don't be afraid to ask butchers or farmers about their procedures. Inquire about how animals are reared, fed, and processed.

**Seasonal Availability:** Be careful of seasonal fluctuations in availability of specific meats and shellfish. This is frequently consistent with sustainable methods.

## 9. Cooking with ethically sourced ingredients

Preparation Techniques

**Simple Cooking Methods:** High-quality meats frequently shine with minimum seasoning and simple cooking techniques such as grilling, roasting, or pan-searing.

**Resting Time:** Let cooked meats rest before slicing to retain juices and improve flavor and texture.

Flavor Pairing

Use fresh herbs, citrus zest, or high-quality oils to enhance the inherent flavors of ethically sourced meats without overwhelming them.

**Cooking Times:** High-quality meats might cook faster due to lower fat content. Use a meat thermometer to guarantee proper doneness without overcooking.

## 10. Storing Quality Meats

**Proper Storage Techniques**

**Refrigeration:** Place fresh meat in the coldest part of your refrigerator (typically in the back) and consume within a few days of purchase.

If you don't plan to use the meat right away, freeze it in airtight packing to avoid freezer burn. Date-labeled parcels make tracking easier.

**Thawing safely**

To avoid bacterial growth, always defrost frozen meat in the refrigerator or under running cold water. Do not thaw at room temperature.

## How to read meat labels and understand phrases like "organic" and "free-range."

Understanding meat labels is critical for making informed decisions regarding the quality and ethical source of your food. Here's a guide to understanding common phrases like "organic" and "free-range."

**1. Organic meat is from animals raised without synthetic pesticides, herbicides, or fertilizers. They also do not receive antibiotics or growth hormones.**

Standards: To be designated organic, farms must follow strict USDA requirements that ensure animals have access to pasture and are fed organic feed. This often leads to greater animal welfare standards and potentially healthier meat.

**2. Definition:** Free-range refers to animals having access to outdoor areas during the day. However, specifics vary greatly depending on country and certification.

USDA Standards: The USDA requires poultry to have access to the outdoors, but it does not specify how much time they must spend outside or the quality of that outdoor space. This indicates that "free-range" does not imply good welfare conditions.

Variability: The word can be misleading; some farms may only offer limited outdoor access, such as little dirt patches rather than beautiful pastures. Always look for additional certificates to provide assurance.

**3. Pasture-Raised:** Animals raised on pasture for a major period of their lives can engage in natural activities.

Certification: There are no common standards for pasture-raised, so seek for third-party certifications like Certified Humane or Animal Welfare. Approved for providing meaningful outdoor access and animal welfare.

**4. Cage-Free Definition:** Cage-free eggs are produced by chickens that are not caged and have free movement within a building or room. However, this does not ensure outdoor access.

Limitations: While cage-free systems are an improvement over caged systems, they may still involve overcrowded conditions, which can cause stress and aggression in hens.

**5. Grass-Fed Definition:** Grass-fed meat originates from animals that eat grass instead of grains. This diet can result in leaner meat containing more omega-3 fatty acids.

Certification: Look for labels that say 100% grass-fed to ensure the animals were never fed grain.

**6. Definition:** Wild-caught seafood is fish and shellfish collected from their natural habitats rather than farms.

Sustainability: Wild-caught choices are frequently regarded as more sustainable, however it is critical to verify sourcing procedures using tools such as the Seafood Watch program.

**7. Additional Terms.**

No Added Hormones/Antibiotics: These phrases imply that no hormones or antibiotics were used during production; nevertheless, it is crucial to note that the use of hormones in chicken is already prohibited in the United States.

Vegetarian-Fed: Although this label implies that hens are fed a vegetarian diet, chickens are naturally omnivorous and may benefit from a diverse diet that includes insects.

# Chapter 7: 60 High-Protein Recipes for Every Meal:

## Breakfasts: High-Protein Recipes

### Steak and eggs.

Begin your day with a protein-rich lunch of steak and eggs. This traditional meal is quick to prepare and will keep you energized all morning.

**Prep time: 10 minutes, Cooking Time: 10 minutes and Serving Size: Two servings**

### Ingredients:

- ❖ 2 thin-cut steaks (4 oz each)
- ❖ 1 teaspoon sea salt.
- ❖ ½ teaspoon black pepper
- ❖ 2 tablespoons avocado oil (divided)
- ❖ Four big eggs.

### Instructions:

- Season the meat with salt and pepper.
- Heat 1 tablespoon avocado oil in a pan over medium-high heat.
- Cook the steaks for about 2 minutes per side, or until desired doneness.
- Remove the steaks from the skillet and allow them to rest.
- In the same skillet, heat the remaining oil and crack the eggs. Cook until the whites have set and the yolks are runny.
- Serve the cut steak with the fried eggs.

**Nutrition Facts**
Calories: About 548 per serving
Protein: Approximately 50g

**Modifications/Substitutes**
Use olive oil instead of avocado oil.
Replace eggs with egg whites for a lower-cholesterol alternative.

# Morning Sausages

These handmade morning sausages are tasty and protein-packed, giving them a fantastic start to the day. They are simple to prepare and may be made in bulk for meal planning.

**Prep time: 10 minutes, Cook time: 15 minutes and 4 serves (8 sausages).**

## Ingredients:
- ❖ 1 pound ground pork or turkey.
- ❖ 1 teaspoon sage.
- ❖ 1 teaspoon thyme.
- ❖ Ingredients: ½ teaspoon salt, ¼ teaspoon black pepper.

## Instructions:
- In a bowl, add all of the ingredients and stir thoroughly.
- Form into tiny patties.
- Cook patties in a skillet over medium heat for about 5 minutes on each side, until browned and cooked through.

**Nutrition Facts**
Calories: Around 200 per serving (2 sausages).
Protein: about 20g

**Modifications/Substitutions**
To create alternative flavor profiles, substitute chicken or beef for pork.
For added flavor, stir in chopped onions or garlic.

# Beany Breakfast Burritos

These beany breakfast burritos are packed in protein and portable, making them excellent for hectic mornings. They're packed with taste and nutrition and will keep you satisfied.

**Prep time: 10 minutes, Cook time: 5 minutes and Serving size: two burritos.**

## Ingredients:
- ❖ 1 whole wheat tortilla.
- ❖ Two huge eggs.
- ❖ 1/2 cup black beans, canned and drained.

❖ Salsa for flavor

**Instructions:**
- Scramble the eggs in a nonstick skillet over medium heat until fully done.
- Warm the tortilla in another pan or microwave.
- Layer the tortilla with black beans and scrambled eggs, followed by salsa and a tight wrap.
- Serve immediately or store in foil for later.

**Nutrition Facts:**
Calories: Around 350 per burrito
Protein: Approximately 22g

**Modifications/Substitutes**
Use egg whites to cut calories.
Replace black beans with pinto or kidney beans.


# Protein Overnight Oats

These protein-rich overnight oats. They are simple to make ahead of time and deliver sustained energy throughout your hectic morning.

**Prep time: 5 minutes, Cooking Time: None (chill overnight) and Serving Size: One serving**

**Ingredients:**
- ❖ 1/2 cup rolled oats.
- ❖ 1/2 cup Greek yogurt.
- ❖ 1/2 cup milk (dairy or plant-based).
- ❖ 1 tablespoon chia seeds.
- ❖ Toppings (berries, nuts) as desired.

**Instructions:**
- In a jar, combine the oats, Greek yogurt, milk, and chia seeds.
- Stir thoroughly to incorporate, and make sure the oats are submerged in liquid.
- Cover and refrigerate overnight.

- Before serving, sprinkle berries or nuts on top.

**Nutrition Facts**
Calories: Around 400 per serving.
Protein: Approximately 25g

**Modifications/Substitutes**
To make it dairy-free, use almond milk instead.
Add protein powder to get an extra protein boost.


# Greek Yogurt Parfait With Nuts

This Greek yogurt parfait is not only tasty, but it also contains protein and healthy fats from almonds. It's a quick breakfast alternative that may be tailored to your preferences.

**Prep time: 5 minutes, Cooking Time: None and Serving Size: One serving.**

## Ingredients:
- 1 cup Greek yogurt, plain or flavored.
- ¼ cup granola
- 2 tablespoons mixed nuts (almonds and walnuts)
- Fresh fruit (berries or bananas) as desired.

## Instructions:
- In a dish or glass, place half of the Greek yogurt on the bottom.
- Place half of the granola and nuts on top.
- Repeat layering with the remaining yogurt, granola, and nuts.
- Prior to serving, top with fresh fruit.

**Nutrition Facts:**
Calories: About 350 per serving.
Protein: about 30g

**Modifications/Substitutes:**
As a vegan option, use dairy-free yogurt.
Replace granola with seeds to reduce carbohydrates.

# Cottage Cheese, Fruit, and Honey

Begin your day with this pleasant and protein-rich cottage cheese dish. It's quick to make and may be personalized using your favorite fruits.

**Prep time: 5 minutes, Cooking Time: None and Serving Size: One serving**

## Ingredients:
- ❖ 1 cup cottage cheese.
- ❖ 1/2 cup mixed fruit (such as berries, bananas, or peaches)
- ❖ 1 tablespoon honey.
- ❖ Optional: Sprinkle cinnamon or nuts for topping.

## Instructions:
- In a bowl, combine the cottage cheese.
- Top with your preferred mixed fruit.
- Drizzle honey on top and, if preferred, sprinkle with cinnamon or nuts.

**Nutrition Facts:**
Calories: around 300.
Protein: Approximately 28g

**Modifications/Substitutes:**
To change up the texture, replace cottage cheese with Greek yogurt.
For a vegan version, substitute maple syrup instead of honey.


# Spinach and Feta Omelette.

This spinach and feta omelet is a simple and high-protein breakfast alternative. It takes less than ten minutes to prepare and is ideal for hectic mornings.

**Prep time: 2 minutes, Cook time: 6 minutes and Serving Size: One serving**

## Ingredients:
- ❖ Two huge eggs.
- ❖ 1 cup fresh spinach, roughly chopped.
- ❖ ¼ cup crumbled feta cheese

❖ 1 teaspoon olive oil.

❖ Add salt and pepper to taste.

## Instructions:

- In a nonstick skillet, heat olive oil over medium heat.
- Sauté the spinach until wilted (approximately 1 minute).
- In a bowl, combine the eggs, salt, and pepper.
- Pour the eggs into the skillet and let them sit for approximately a minute.
- Sprinkle feta on one half of the omelet and fold the other half over it.
- Cook for one another minute until completely set, then serve.

**Nutrition Facts:**
Calories: Around 250
Protein: Approximately 20g

**Modifications/Substitutes;**
To make a lower-calorie variation, substitute egg whites.
To change the flavor, substitute goat cheese for feta.

## Smoked Salmon and Avocado Toast.

This smoked salmon and avocado toast is not only tasty, but also strong in protein and healthy fats. It's a simple but tasty breakfast option.

**Prep time: 5 minutes, Cooking Time: None and Serving Size: One serving**

## Ingredients:

❖ 1 piece whole-grain bread, toasted

❖ 1/2 avocado (mashed)

❖ 2 ounces smoked salmon

❖ Add salt and pepper to taste.

## Instructions:

- Toast a slice of whole grain bread.
- Spread the mashed avocado on top of the toast.
- Layer the avocado with smoked salmon.

- Season with salt, pepper, and optional lemon juice or capers.
- Optional garnishes include lemon juice and capers.

**Nutrition Facts**
Calories: Around 350
Protein: Approximately 25g

**Modifications/Substitutes**
To make an alternative spread, substitute cream cheese for avocado.
Replace smoked salmon with canned tuna for a different protein source.

# Peanut Butter Banana Smoothie

A protein-rich breakfast alternative. It's ideal for busy mornings when you need something nourishing on-the-go.

**Prep time: 5 minutes, Cooking Time: None and Serving Size: One serving**

## Ingredients:
- One ripe banana.
- 2 tablespoons peanut butter.
- 1 cup milk, either dairy or plant-based.
- Optional: Ice cubes for a thicker smoothie.

## Instructions:
- In a blender, combine the banana, peanut butter, milk, and ice cubes, if desired.
- Blend until smooth.
- Pour into a glass and drink immediately.

**Nutrition Facts**
Calories: Around 400
Protein: Approximately 15g

**Modifications/Substitutes**
To change up the nut flavor, substitute almond butter for peanut butter.
Add protein powder to get an extra protein boost.

# Quinoa Breakfast Bowl with Almonds.

This quinoa breakfast bowl is a nutritious way to start the day, full of protein from quinoa and healthy fats from almonds. It's easy to plan ahead of time!

**Preparation Time: 10 minutes (including overnight soak if desired), Cook time: 15 minutes and Serving Size: One serving.**

## Ingredients:
- ½ cup cooked quinoa.
- 1/2 cup almond milk (or any milk)
- 2 tablespoons sliced almonds.
- 1 tablespoon honey or maple syrup.
- Optional toppings include fresh fruit or chia seeds.

## Instructions:
- In a mixing dish, add cooked quinoa and almond milk. Stir thoroughly.
- Drizzle honey or maple syrup over top.
- Sprinkle with sliced almonds and any desired toppings.
- Serve either warm or cold.

**Nutrition Facts**
Calories: Around 350
Protein: about 12g

**Modifications/Substitutes**
To add diversity, substitute any other nuts or seeds for the almonds.
For a different grain foundation, use oats instead of quinoa.

# Egg Muffins with Vegetables and Cheese

These egg muffins are an excellent high-protein breakfast choice that can be made ahead of time. They're packed with veggies and cheese, making them ideal for hectic mornings!

**Prep time: 10 minutes, Cook time: 20 minutes and Serving size: six muffins.**

## Ingredients:
- Six big eggs.

- ❖ 1 cup chopped spinach
- ❖ 1/2 cup diced bell pepper.
- ❖ 1/2 cup sliced onion.
- ❖ 1/2 cup shredded cheese (either cheddar or your preferred type)
- ❖ Add salt and pepper to taste.

## Instructions:

- Preheat the oven to 350°F/175°C and oil a muffin pan.
- In a mixing dish, whisk the eggs and season with salt and pepper.
- Add the chopped spinach, bell pepper, onion, and cheese to the egg mixture.
- Pour the mixture equally into the muffin tin.
- Bake for 18-20 minutes, or until the muffins have set.
- Allow to cool somewhat before removing from the tin.

**Nutrition Facts**
Calories: About 120 per muffin
Protein: Approximately 10g

**Modifications/Substitutes**
To make a lower-calorie variation, substitute egg whites.
Add cooked bacon or sausage for added flavor.

# Chia Seed Pudding with Berries

This protein-rich breakfast is both delicious and nutritious. It's simple to cook and may be started the night before for a quick morning supper.

**Prep time: 5 minutes, Cooking Time: None (chill overnight) and Serving Size: One serving**

## Ingredients:

- ❖ ¼ cup Chia seeds
- ❖ 1 cup almond milk (or other milk)
- ❖ 1 tablespoon honey or maple syrup.
- ❖ 1/2 cup mixed berries, fresh or frozen.

## Instructions:

- In a bowl or jar, combine the chia seeds, almond milk, and honey.
- Stir well to prevent clumps.
- Cover and refrigerate overnight.
- Stir again in the morning, then top with mixed berries before serving.

**Nutrition Facts**
Calories: around 300.
Protein: Approximately 10g

**Modifications/Substitutes**
Use coconut milk to add a tropical flavor.
For a vegan version, use agave syrup instead of honey.

## Breakfast Tacos and Scrambled Eggs

These morning tacos with scrambled eggs are quick to make and high in protein. They are ideal for a hearty breakfast that you may tailor to your preferences!

**Prep time: 10 minutes, Cooking Time: 10 minutes and Serving Size: four tacos.**

### Ingredients:
- Four big eggs.
- 4 tiny tortillas (corn or wheat).
- ½ sliced avocado.
- ¼ cup shredded cheese (either cheddar or Mexican blend).
- Add salt and pepper to taste.
- Optional toppings include salsa and cilantro.

### Instructions:
- In a bowl, combine the eggs, salt, and pepper.
- Heat a nonstick skillet over medium heat, then scramble the eggs until just set.
- Warm the tortillas in another skillet or microwave.
- Fill each tortilla with scrambled eggs, then top with cheese, avocado, and any other desired toppings.

**Nutrition Facts**

Calories: About 250 per taco

Protein: Approximately 15g

**Modifications/Substitutes**

For more protein, add cooked bacon or sausage.

Use egg whites for a lighter option.

# High Protein Pancakes

These high-protein pancakes are fluffy and tasty, making them a wonderful way to begin your day! They're simple to prepare and can be topped with your favorite fruits.

**Prep time: 5 minutes, Cooking Time: 10 minutes and Serving size: two pancakes.**

## Ingredients

- ❖ 1 cup oats, mixed into flour
- ❖ 1 scoop of protein powder, either vanilla or unflavored.
- ❖ One huge egg.
- ❖ 3/4 cup milk (dairy or plant-based)
- ❖ Optional toppings include maple syrup and berries.

## Instructions:

- In a mixing dish, combine oat flour, protein powder, egg, and milk until smooth.
- To make pancakes, heat a nonstick skillet over medium heat and pour batter in.
- Cook until bubbles form on the surface, then flip and cook until golden brown on both sides.
- Serve warm with your preferred toppings.

**Nutrition Facts**

Calories: about 300 for two pancakes.

Protein: Approximately 25g

**Modifications/Substitutes**

To make a gluten-free variation, substitute almond flour for oat flour.

For more taste, mix in some mashed banana or pumpkin puree.

# Savory oatmeal with a poached egg.

This savory oatmeal with poached egg is a unique high-protein breakfast that is both full and nutritious. It's ideal for individuals who prefer a hearty start to the day!

**Prep time: 5 minutes, Cooking Time: 10 minutes and Serving Size: One serving**

## Ingredients:
- ❖ 1/2 cup rolled oats.
- ❖ 1 cup water or broth.
- ❖ Salt to taste.
- ❖ One huge egg.
- ❖ Optional toppings include spinach, cheese, and spicy sauce.

## Instructions:
- Bring a pot of water or broth to a boil; then add the oats and salt.
- Reduce the heat and cook the oats for about 5 minutes.
- Meanwhile, poach the egg in simmering water until the whites have set (approximately 3 minutes).
- Serve oatmeal in a bowl, topped with the poached egg and any other toppings.

**Nutrition Facts**
Calories: Around 250
Protein: about 14g.

**Modifications/Substitutes**
To change things up, substitute quinoa for oats.
Sauté vegetables for added nutrients.

# Lunches: Portable and Filling Meals

## Meatballs with vegetables.

These meatballs with vegetables are a tasty and protein-rich lunch alternative. They are simple to prepare and may be served hot or cold, making them ideal for meal prep!

**Prep time: 15 minutes, Cook time: 20 minutes and Serving Size: Four servings**

## Ingredients:
- ❖ 1 pound ground beef or turkey.
- ❖ 1 cup breadcrumbs.
- ❖ One huge egg.
- ❖ 1 teaspoon Italian seasoning.
- ❖ 1 cup mixed vegetables (carrots, bell peppers, and zucchini).
- ❖ Add salt and pepper to taste.

## Instructions:
- Preheat the oven to 400 °F (200 °C).
- In a bowl, combine the ground beef, breadcrumbs, egg, Italian seasoning, salt, and pepper.
- Form the mixture into meatballs approximately the size of a golf ball.
- Place the meatballs on a baking pan and bake for 15-20 minutes, or until well cooked.
- Steam or sauté the mixed vegetables until tender.
- Serve the meatballs with vegetables on the side.

**Nutrition Facts**
Calories: About 350 per serving.
Protein: Approximately 30g

**Modifications/Substitutes**
Use ground chicken or pork instead of beef or turkey.
For added taste, add shredded cheese to the meatball mixture.

# Hearty salad with grilled chicken.

This substantial salad with grilled chicken is full of protein and fresh ingredients. It's a filling dish that's simple to make and ideal for lunch on the road.

**Prep time: 10 minutes, Cook time: 15 minutes and Serving Size: Two servings**

## Ingredients:
- ❖ 2 boneless, skinless chicken breasts.
- ❖ 4 cups mixed greens (spinach and romaine)
- ❖ 1 cup cherry tomatoes, halved
- ❖ ½ cucumber, sliced
- ❖ ¼ cup crumbled feta cheese
- ❖ To season, combine olive oil, salt, and pepper.

## Instructions:
- Preheat the grill or skillet to medium-high heat.
- Season the chicken breasts with olive oil, salt, and pepper.
- Grill the chicken for 6-7 minutes per side, or until thoroughly done.
- Let the chicken rest for a few minutes before slicing.
- In a large bowl, combine the mixed greens, cherry tomatoes, cucumber, and feta.
- Drizzle olive oil over the salad and top with grilled chicken slices.

**Nutrition Facts**
Calories: Around 400 per serving.
Protein: Approximately 35g

**Modifications/Substitutes**
To make a vegetarian dish, substitute tofu or chickpeas for the chicken.
Replace feta cheese for goat cheese for a different flavor.

# Quinoa Salad With Chickpeas

This quinoa salad with chickpeas is strong in protein and incredibly filling. It's an excellent lunch choice that can be prepared ahead of time and eaten cold.

**Prep time: 10 minutes, Cook time: 15 minutes and Serving Size: Four servings**

## Ingredients:
- ❖ 1 cup quinoa, uncooked
- ❖ 1 can chickpeas, drained and rinsed.
- ❖ 1 bell pepper, diced
- ❖ ½ red onion, chopped
- ❖ ¼ cup parsley, chopped
- ❖ Juice from 1 lemon
- ❖ Add olive oil, salt, and pepper to taste.

## Instructions:
- Cook the quinoa according to the package directions and let it cool.
- In a large mixing bowl, add cooked quinoa, chickpeas, bell pepper, red onion, and parsley.
- Drizzle with lemon juice and olive oil, then season with salt and pepper.
- Toss everything until thoroughly combined.

**Nutrition Facts**
Calories: Around 250 per serving.
Protein: Approximately 12g

**Modifications/Substitutes**
For a creamy texture, add chopped avocado.
Replace chickpeas with black beans or kidney beans.

# Turkey and Spinach Wraps

These turkey and spinach wraps are a quick, high-protein lunch alternative that is simple to prepare and ideal for packing in a lunchbox.

**Prep time: 5 minutes, Cooking Time: None and Serving Size: Two wraps.**

## Ingredients:
- ❖ Four whole wheat tortillas.
- ❖ 8 ounces sliced turkey breast
- ❖ 2 cups of fresh spinach leaves.

* ½ avocado, sliced
* Mustard or hummus to spread

## Instructions:
* Lay out the tortillas on a level surface.
* Spread mustard or hummus on each tortilla.
* Layer the turkey pieces, spinach leaves, and avocado on top.
* Roll each tortilla tightly and cut in half to serve.

## Nutrition Facts
Calories: Around 300 per wrap
Protein: Approximately 25g

## Modifications/Substitutes
For added diversity, substitute grilled chicken for turkey.
For added crunch, mix in sliced cucumbers or bell peppers.

## Lentil Soup With Ham

This lentil soup with ham is comforting and protein-rich. It's ideal for a cold-weather lunch and may be prepared ahead of time for easy meal planning.

**Prep time: 10 minutes, Cook time: 30 minutes and Serving Size: Four servings**

## Ingredients:
* 1 cup lentils, washed.
* 4 cups vegetable or chicken broth.
* 1 cup of diced ham.
* 1 carrot, diced.
* 1 celery stalk, diced.
* Add salt and pepper to taste.

## Instructions:
* In a large pot over medium heat, add the lentils, stock, ham, carrots, and celery.

- Bring to a boil, then reduce to a simmer for 30 minutes, or until the lentils are cooked.
- Season with salt and pepper before serving.

**Nutrition Facts**
Calories: About 350 per serving.
Protein: Approximately 25g

**Modifications/Substitutes**
For more taste, use smoked sausage instead of ham.
Add spinach or kale near the end of the cooking process for added nutrition.

# Chicken Caesar Salad

This Chicken Caesar Salad is a traditional high-protein meal that features juicy grilled chicken, crisp romaine lettuce, and handmade croutons. It's simple to cook and ideal for a hearty meal.

**Prep time: 15 minutes, Cook time: 25 minutes and Serving Size: Four servings**

## Ingredients;
- 1 pound boneless, skinless chicken breasts.
- 14 ounces romaine lettuce (chopped)
- 1 1/2 cups grated Parmesan cheese
- ¾ cup olive oil, split
- 3 cloves of garlic, minced
- 1 lemon, juiced.
- 2 teaspoons Worcestershire sauce.
- Add salt and pepper to taste.
- For croutons:
- 8 pieces of bread, cubed
- 1/4 cup olive oil.
- Salt to taste.

## Instructions:
- Marinate the chicken in balsamic vinegar, olive oil, salt, and pepper.
- Grill the chicken for about 6 minutes per side, or until well done.

- In a large mixing bowl, combine the romaine, olive oil, minced garlic, lemon juice, Worcestershire sauce, salt, and pepper.
- Add grated Parmesan cheese and blend thoroughly.
- Slice the grilled chicken and arrange it on top of the salad.
- To make croutons, mix bread cubes with olive oil and toast in a skillet until brown.
- Before serving, top the salad with croutons and more cheese.

**Nutrition Facts**
Calories: Around 450 per serving
Protein: Approximately 40g

**Modifications/Substitutes**
To add a seafood twist, use grilled shrimp instead of chicken.
To change up the flavor, replace the Parmesan with feta cheese.

## Tuna Salad, Lettuce Wraps

Tuna Salad Lettuce Wraps are a protein-rich, light lunch choice. They are simple to prepare and ideal for on-the-go dinners!

Prep time: 10 minutes, Cooking Time: None and Serving Size: Two servings

**Ingredients:**
- 1 can (5 oz) tuna, drained
- 1/4 cup Greek yogurt or mayonnaise.
- 1 celery stalk, diced.
- 1 tablespoon Dijon mustard.
- Add salt and pepper to taste.
- lettuce leaves (to wrap)

**Instructions:**
- In a bowl, combine drained tuna, Greek yogurt or mayonnaise, diced celery, Dijon mustard, salt, and pepper.
- Spoon the tuna mixture onto big lettuce leaves.
- Roll up the leaves into bundles and serve immediately.

**Nutrition Facts**
Calories: Around 250 per serving.
Protein: Approximately 30g

**Modifications/Substitutes**
For added diversity, use canned salmon for tuna.
Add diced pickles or onions for some added crunch.

# Beef and Broccoli Stir-fry

This beef and broccoli stir-fry is a simple and protein-rich lunch choice. It tastes great and takes less than 30 minutes to prepare!

**Prep time: 10 minutes, Cook time: 15 minutes and Serving Size: Four servings**

## Ingredients:
- ❖ 1 pound beef sirloin (sliced thinly)
- ❖ 4 cups broccoli florets.
- ❖ 3 tablespoons soy sauce.
- ❖ 2 tablespoons of oyster sauce (optional).
- ❖ 2 cloves of garlic, minced
- ❖ 1 teaspoon ginger (minced)
- ❖ Olive oil for cooking.

## Instructions:
- Heat olive oil in a large skillet over medium-high heat.
- Cook the sliced meat until browned, then remove from the skillet.
- In the same skillet, combine the broccoli, garlic, and ginger; stir cook until soft.
- Return the steak to the skillet, then add the soy sauce and oyster sauce. Stir well.
- Cook for an additional minute, until thoroughly heated.

**Nutrition Facts**
Calories: About 350 per serving.
Protein: Approximately 30g

**Modifications/Substitutes**

For a variety of protein options, substitute chicken or tofu for beef.

Add bell peppers or snap peas for added vegetables.

# Mediterranean Chickpea Bowl

This Mediterranean Chickpea Bowl is a colorful and nutritious lunch choice high in protein from chickpea. It's ideal for meal planning and a fast lunch!

**Prep time: 10 minutes, Cooking Time: None and Serving Size: Four servings**

## Ingredients:

- ❖ 1 can (15 oz) chickpeas, drained and rinsed.
- ❖ 1 cup cherry tomatoes, halved
- ❖ ½ cucumber, diced
- ❖ ¼ red onion, chopped
- ❖ 1/2 cup crumbled feta cheese.
- ❖ Juice from 1 lemon
- ❖ Add olive oil, salt, and pepper to taste.

## Instructions:

- In a large mixing basin, add chickpeas, cherry tomatoes, cucumber, red onion, and feta cheese.
- Drizzle with lemon juice and olive oil, then season with salt and pepper.
- Toss everything until thoroughly combined.

**Nutrition Facts**

Calories: Around 300 per serving.

Protein: Approximately 15g

**Modifications/Substitutes**

To change the flavor, substitute goat cheese for feta.

For a more Mediterranean flavor, add olives or roasted red peppers.

# Shrimp and Avocado Salad

This Shrimp and Avocado Salad is light but filling, making it a fantastic high-protein lunch choice. It's fresh, tasty, and simple to cook!

**Prep time: 10 minutes, Cook Time: None (when using pre-cooked shrimp) and Serving Size: Two servings**

## Ingredients:

- ❖ 8 ounces cooked shrimp, peeled and deveined.
- ❖ 1 avocado, diced.
- ❖ 2 cups mixed greens.
- ❖ Juice of one lime
- ❖ Add olive oil, salt, and pepper to taste.

## Instructions:

- In a bowl, add cooked shrimp and diced avocado.
- Drizzle with lime juice and olive oil, then season with salt and pepper.
- Serve on a bed of mixed greens.

**Nutrition Facts**
Calories: About 350 per serving.
Protein: Approximately 25g

**Modifications/Substitutes**
For added diversity, use crab meat for shrimp.
For added freshness, add cherry tomatoes or cucumber.

# BBQ Pulled Pork Sandwiches.

These BBQ Pulled Pork Sandwiches are soft and tasty, ideal for a high-protein lunch. They're simple to make in the slow cooker and ideal for meal prep or entertaining!

**Prep time: 10 minutes, Cooking Time: 8 hours (slow cooker) and Serving size: four sandwiches.**

## Ingredients:

- ❖ 3 pound boneless pork shoulder

* 1 teaspoon salt.
* ½ teaspoon black pepper
* 2 cups of low-sodium chicken broth.
* 2 tablespoons liquid smoke.
* 3 cups BBQ sauce (plus extra to serve)
* 4 hamburger buns.

## Instructions:

- Season the pork with salt and pepper.
- Put the meat in a slow cooker with broth and liquid smoke.
- Cook on low for 8 hours, until the meat is tender.
- Shred the meat using forks and combine with the BBQ sauce.
- Serve on buns with more barbecue sauce.

**Nutrition Facts**
Calories: About 670 per sandwich
Protein: Approximately 34g

**Modifications/Substitutes**
For a lighter option, choose chicken or turkey.
To add extra crunch, top the sandwich with coleslaw.

# Egg Salad with Whole Grain Bread

This Egg Salad on Whole Grain Bread is a classic high-protein meal that is simple to prepare and portable. It's creamy, delicious, and flavorful!

**Prep time: 10 minutes, Cooking Time: None and Serving Size: Two servings**

## Ingredients:

* 4 large eggs (hard cooked)
* 1/4 cup Greek yogurt or mayonnaise.
* 1 teaspoon Dijon mustard.
* Add salt and pepper to taste.
* 4 pieces of whole grain bread.

## Instructions:

- Peel and cut the hard-boiled eggs.
- In a bowl, combine eggs, Greek yogurt or mayonnaise, Dijon mustard, salt, and pepper.
- Spread the egg salad over whole grain bread and create sandwiches.

**Nutrition Facts**

Calories: Around 300 per serving.
Protein: Approximately 20g

**Modifications/Substitutes**

Use avocado instead of mayonnaise for a healthier alternative.
Add diced celery or pickles for an added crunch.

## Falafel Wraps With Tahini Sauce

These Falafel Wraps with Tahini Sauce are a tasty, high-protein vegetarian lunch choice. They are flavorful and ideal for on-the-go meals!

**Prep time: 15 minutes, Cook for 10 minutes (if using pre-made falafel) and Serving Size: Two wraps.**

## Ingredients:

- ❖ 1 cup cooked falafel, either store-bought or homemade.
- ❖ Two whole wheat tortillas or pita bread
- ❖ 1 cup mixed greens.
- ❖ ½ cucumber, sliced
- ❖ ¼ cup tahini sauce

## Instructions:

- Warm tortillas or pita bread.
- Put falafel on each wrap.
- Top with mixed greens and cucumber slices, then sprinkle with tahini sauce.
- Roll the wraps securely and serve.

**Nutrition Facts**

Calories: roughly 400 per wrap

Protein: Approximately 15g
**Modifications/Substitutes**
To change up the flavor, substitute hummus for tahini sauce.
For more vegetables, add sliced tomatoes or bell peppers.

## Grilled Chicken with Quinoa Bowl

This Grilled Chicken and Quinoa Bowl is a high-protein, healthful, and simple lunch option. It's ideal for meal prep and may be tailored to your preferences!

**Prep time: 10 minutes, Cook time: 20 minutes and Serving size: two bowls.**

## Ingredients:

- ❖ 1 pound boneless, skinless chicken breast.
- ❖ 1 cup quinoa, uncooked
- ❖ 2 cups of water or broth.
- ❖ Add salt and pepper to taste.
- ❖ Optional toppings include avocado, cherry tomatoes, and spinach.

## Instructions:

- Cook quinoa according to package directions and set aside.
- Season chicken breasts with salt and pepper and grill until done (approximately 6 minutes per side).
- Slice the grilled chicken.
- In bowls, combine quinoa, cut chicken, and any preferred toppings.

**Nutrition Facts**
Calories: About 450 per bowl
Protein: Approximately 40g

**Modifications/Substitutes**
To make a vegetarian dish, substitute tofu for the chicken.
Replace quinoa with brown rice or farro.

## Stuffed peppers with ground turkey.

Stuffed Peppers with Ground Turkey are a healthy, high-protein lunch choice that is both colorful and delicious. They're easy to prepare ahead of time and ideal for meal planning!

**Prep time: 15 minutes, Cook time: 30 minutes and Serving Size: Four Stuffed Peppers**

## Ingredients:

- ❖ 4 bell peppers, any color.
- ❖ 1 pound ground turkey
- ❖ 1 cup cooked rice, brown or white.
- ❖ 1 can of chopped tomatoes (14 ounces)
- ❖ Add salt and pepper to taste.

## Instructions:

- Preheat the oven to 375° Fahrenheit (190° Celsius).
- Cut the tops of bell peppers and remove the seeds.
- In a skillet, brown the ground turkey; then add the cooked rice, diced tomatoes, salt, and pepper.
- Stuff each pepper with turkey mixture.
- Place the filled peppers in a baking dish, cover with foil, and bake for approximately 30 minutes.

**Nutrition Facts**

Calories: Around 300 per stuffed pepper.

Protein: Approximately 25g

**Modifications/Substitutes**

Use ground beef or chicken instead of turkey.

For added nourishment, combine the stuffing with black beans or corn.

# Dinners: Flavorful Variety

## Roasted Lamb

This Roasted Lamb is a luscious and tasty dish suitable for a special dinner. It's packed in protein and can be paired with your favorite sides to make a complete dinner.

**Prep time: 15 minutes, Cooking time: 1 hour 30 minutes and Serving Size: Four servings**

### Ingredients:
- ❖ 2 pound leg of lamb
- ❖ 4 garlic cloves (sliced)
- ❖ 2 tbsp fresh rosemary, chopped
- ❖ 2 tablespoons of olive oil.
- ❖ Add salt and pepper to taste.
- ❖ Optional: vegetables (carrots, potatoes) to roast.

### Instructions:
- Preheat the oven to 375° Fahrenheit (190° Celsius).
- Make small slits in the lamb, then insert garlic pieces and rosemary.
- Coat the lamb with olive oil, salt, and pepper.
- Place the lamb in a roasting pan, surrounded by veggies if desired.
- Roast for approximately 1 hour and 30 minutes, or until the internal temperature reaches 145°F (medium rare).
- Rest for 10 minutes before slicing.

**Nutrition Facts**
Calories: Around 450 per serving
Protein: Approximately 40g

**Modifications/Substitutes**
A rack of lamb makes a more elegant appearance.
For a distinct flavor, choose thyme or oregano instead of rosemary.

# BBQ brisket

This barbecue brisket is tender, juicy, and full of flavor. It's ideal for feeding a large group or planning meals for the week ahead!

**Prep time: 10 minutes, Cooking Time: 8 hours (slow cooker) and Serving Size: 6 Servings**

## Ingredients:

- ❖ 3 pound beef brisket
- ❖ 1 cup BBQ sauce, homemade or store-bought.
- ❖ 2 tablespoons Worcestershire sauce.
- ❖ 1 tablespoon brown sugar.
- ❖ Add salt and pepper to taste.

## Instructions:

- Season the brisket with salt and pepper.
- Place the brisket in a slow cooker; add the BBQ sauce and Worcestershire sauce.
- Cook on low for approximately 8 hours, or until tender.
- Brisket should be removed from the cooker and allowed to rest before slicing against the grain.

**Nutrition Facts**
Calories: Around 500 per serving.
Protein: Approximately 40g

**Modifications/Substitutes**
To change up the flavor, use pork shoulder instead of brisket.
To improve the rub, add spices such as paprika or garlic powder.

# Stir-Fried Tofu with Vegetables

Stir-Fried Tofu and Veggies is a quick and healthy meal choice that's strong in protein and full of colorful vegetables. It's ideal for busy weeknights!

**Prep time: 10 minutes, Cooking Time: 10 minutes and Serving Size: Four servings**

**Ingredients:**

- ❖ 14 ounces firm tofu (cubed)
- ❖ 2 cups of mixed vegetables (bell peppers, broccoli, and carrots).
- ❖ 3 tablespoons soy sauce.
- ❖ 1 tablespoon sesame oil.
- ❖ 2 cloves of garlic, minced
- ❖ Optional: Sesame seeds for garnish.

**Instructions:**

- Heat the sesame oil in a large skillet over medium-high heat.
- Add the cubed tofu and heat until golden brown on all sides.
- Stir-fry the mixed vegetables and garlic until they are soft.
- Pour in the soy sauce and stir to coat evenly.
- Serve hot and garnish with sesame seeds if preferred.

**Nutrition Facts**

Calories: Around 250 per serving.
Protein: Approximately 20g

**Modifications/Substitutes**

Use tempeh instead of tofu for a firmer texture.
Replace soy sauce with tamari for a gluten-free version.

## Herb-crusted salmon filets

These herb-crusted salmon filets are not only tasty, but also high in protein and healthy fats. They provide for a nice but simple dinner alternative!

**Prep time: 10 minutes, Cook time: 15 minutes and Serving Size: Four servings**

**Ingredients:**

- ❖ 4 salmon filets, 6 ounces each.
- ❖ 2 tablespoons Dijon mustard.
- ❖ ½ cup breadcrumbs

❖ Fresh parsley, chopped (¼ cup)

❖ Add salt and pepper to taste.

**Instructions:**

- Preheat the oven to 400° F (200° C).
- Arrange the salmon filets on a baking pan lined with parchment paper.
- Spread Dijon mustard on each filet.
- In a bowl, combine the breadcrumbs, parsley, salt, and pepper; press onto the salmon filets.
- Bake for 12-15 minutes, or until the salmon flakes easily with a fork.

**Nutrition Facts**

Calories: About 350 per serving.

Protein: Approximately 30g

**Modifications/Substitutes**

If you like, you can substitute trout or tilapia.

For a crunchier texture, replace breadcrumbs with crushed nuts.

## Chicken Thighs With Garlic And Lemon

These chicken thighs with garlic and lemon are juicy and flavorful! This high-protein dish is simple to prepare and ideal for a family meal.

**Prep time: 10 minutes, Cook time: 30 minutes and Serving Size: Four servings**

**Ingredients**

- ❖ 4 bone-in chicken thighs (with skin on)
- ❖ Juice from 1 lemon
- ❖ Zest from 1 lemon
- ❖ 4 cloves garlic, minced
- ❖ Add salt and pepper to taste.
- ❖ Fresh parsley for garnish.

**Instructions:**

- Preheat the oven to 425° Fahrenheit (220° Celsius).

- In a bowl, combine lemon juice, zest, minced garlic, salt, and pepper.
- Place the chicken thighs in a baking dish and pour the lemon mixture over.
- Bake for about 30 minutes, or until the chicken is well cooked (internal temperature of 165°F).
- Garnish with fresh parsley before serving.

**Nutrition Facts**
Calories: Around 400 per serving.
Protein: Approximately 35g

**Modifications/Substitutes**
Boneless chicken thighs are ideal for quick cooking.
For a variety of flavors, substitute lime or orange juice in place of lemon.

## Stuffed Portobello Mushrooms With Sausage

**Prep time: 15 minutes, Cook time: 25 minutes and Serving Size: 4**

## Ingredients:
- ❖ 4 huge Portobello mushrooms
- ❖ 1 cup Italian sausage, cooked and crumbled
- ❖ 1/2 cup ricotta cheese.
- ❖ 1/4 cup grated parmesan cheese.
- ❖ 1/2 cup chopped spinach.
- ❖ Add salt and pepper to taste.

## Instructions:
- Preheat the oven to 375° Fahrenheit (190° Celsius).
- Remove the stems from the mushrooms and lay the caps on a baking sheet.
- In a bowl, combine the sausage, ricotta, Parmesan, spinach, salt, and pepper.
- Stuff the mixture into the mushroom tops.
- Bake for 20 minutes, until the mushrooms are soft.

**Nutrition facts:**
Each serving contains around 220 calories and
20g of protein.

## Grilled shrimp skewers with vegetables.

**Prep time: 10 minutes, Cooking Time: 10 minutes and Serving Size: 4**

### Ingredients:
- ❖ 1 pound shrimp, peeled and deveined.
- ❖ Two bell peppers, chopped
- ❖ 1 zucchini, sliced
- ❖ 2 tablespoons of olive oil.
- ❖ Add salt and pepper to taste.

### Instructions:
- Preheat the grill for medium-high heat.
- Toss the shrimp and vegetables with olive oil, salt, and pepper.
- Thread shrimp and vegetables onto skewers.
- Grill the shrimp for about 5 minutes on each side, until they are opaque.

**Nutrition facts:**
Each serving contains around 180 calories and
25g of protein.

**Modifications/Substitutes:**
Use chicken or tofu instead of shrimp.

## Classic meatloaf with mashed potatoes.

**Prep time: 15 minutes, Cook time: one hour and Serving Size: 6**

### Ingredients:
- ❖ 1 pound ground beef or turkey.
- ❖ 1 cup breadcrumbs.
- ❖ 1 egg
- ❖ 1/2 cup minced onion.

❖ 1/4 cup ketchup.

**Instructions:**
- Preheat the oven to 350° Fahrenheit (175° Celsius).
- Combine all of the ingredients in a bowl.
- Form into a loaf and place in a baking dish.
- Bake for approximately 60 minutes, or until thoroughly cooked.

**Nutrition facts:**
Each serving contains around 300 calories and
30g of protein.

**Modifications:**
For a gluten-free version, replace breadcrumbs with oats.

## Thai Red Curry Chicken

**Prep time: 10 minutes, Cook time: 20 minutes and Serving Size: 4**

**Ingredients:**
- ❖ 1 pound chicken breast, cut
- ❖ 1 can coconut milk (14 ounces)
- ❖ 2 tablespoons of red curry paste.
- ❖ 1 cup bell peppers, sliced
- ❖ Fresh basil for garnish.

**Instructions:**
- Heat a pan over medium heat; add the chicken and cook until browned.
- Stir in the curry paste and coconut milk, then simmer for about 10 minutes.
- Add the bell peppers and simmer until tender.
- Serve garnished with fresh basil.

**Nutrition facts:**
Each serving contains around 350 calories and 28g of protein.

**Modifications/Substitutes:**

Vegetarians can use tofu in place of meat.

# Ratatouille with Grilled Sausages

**Prep time: 15 minutes, Cook time: 30 minutes and Serving Size: 4**

## Ingredients:
- ❖ One zucchini, diced
- ❖ One eggplant, chopped
- ❖ 1 bell pepper, diced
- ❖ Two tomatoes, chopped
- ❖ Olive oil for sautéing.

## Instructions:
- In a skillet, heat the olive oil and sauté the zucchini, eggplant, and bell pepper until tender (10 minutes).
- Cook for an additional 10 minutes, until everything is tender.
- Serve with grilled sausages for extra protein.

**Nutritional information:**
Approximately 200 calories (without sausages); protein content varies depending on sausage choice.

**Modifications:**
For more protein, add lentils or other seasonal veggies that are available.

# Snacks and sides.

## Jerky (beef or Turkey)

**Prep time: 15 minutes, Cooking Time: 4-6 hours and Serving Size: One ounce.**

### Ingredients:
- ❖ 1 pound meat or turkey, thinly sliced
- ❖ 1/4 cup soy sauce.
- ❖ 1 tablespoon of Worcestershire sauce.
- ❖ 1 teaspoon of garlic powder.
- ❖ 1 teaspoon of onion powder.
- ❖ 1 teaspoon of black pepper.

### Instructions:
- Marinate the beef in soy and Worcestershire sauces with spices for at least 4 hours.
- Preheat the dehydrator to 160°F (70°C).
- Place the pork slices in a single layer and dehydrate for 4-6 hours until dry.

**Nutritional information:**
Approximately 10g protein per ounce.

**Modifications/Substitutes:**
Use low-sodium soy sauce for a healthier alternative.

## Bone broth

**Prep time: 10 minutes, Cooking Time: 12-24 hours and Serving size: one cup.**

### Ingredients:
- ❖ 2 pound bones (beef, chicken, or turkey)
- ❖ Two carrots, chopped.
- ❖ Two celery stalks, chopped
- ❖ One onion, quartered
- ❖ 2 teaspoons of apple cider vinegar.

❖ Water to cover.

## Instructions:
- Place the bones and vegetables in a big pot or slow cooker.
- Add vinegar and cover with water.
- Simmer on low for 12-24 hours, scraping the froth as needed.

**Nutrition Facts:**
Each cup contains around 10g of protein.

**Modifications/Substitutes:**
For added taste, add herbs like thyme or bay leaves.

# Vegetable Stir-Fry

**Prep time: 10 minutes, Cook time: 15 minutes and Serving size: two cups.**

## Ingredients:
- ❖ 2 cups of mixed vegetables (carrots, bell peppers, broccoli)
- ❖ 1 cup of cooked chicken or tofu.
- ❖ 2 tablespoons of soy sauce.
- ❖ 1 tablespoon of olive oil.
- ❖ Optional: Sesame seeds for garnish.

## Instructions:
- In a medium-sized pan, heat the olive oil.
- Stir-fry the vegetables for approximately 5 minutes.
- Add the chicken or tofu and soy sauce, and simmer until heated through.

**Nutrition Facts:**
Each serving of chicken has approximately 20g of protein.

**Modifications:**
Substitute whatever vegetables you desire.

# Chia Seed Pudding.

**Prep time: 5 minutes, Cooking Time: None and Serving size: one cup.**

## Ingredients:

- ❖ 1/4 cup chia seeds.
- ❖ 1 cup almond milk (or other milk)
- ❖ 1 tablespoon honey or maple syrup.
- ❖ Optional toppings include fruits and nuts.

## Instructions:

- Combine the chia seeds, milk, and sweetener in a bowl.
- Refrigerate for at least 4 hours or overnight to thicken.
- Serve with the preferred toppings.

**Nutrition facts:**

Each serving contains approximately 6g of protein.

**Modifications:**

To change the flavor, use coconut milk.


# Hard-boiled Eggs

**Prep time: 5 minutes, Cooking Time: 10 minutes and Serving Size: Two eggs.**

## Ingredients:

- ❖ Eggs (as many as desired).

## Instructions:

- Place the eggs in a pot and cover with water.
- Bring to a boil, then cover and remove from the heat.
- Allow to settle for approximately 10 minutes before chilling in ice water.

**Nutrition Facts:**

Each egg contains around 6g of protein.

**Modifications/Substitutes:**

For added flavor, season with salt and pepper.

# Roasted chickpeas.

**Prep time: 10 minutes, Cook time: 30 minutes and Serving Size: Four servings**

## Ingredients:
- ❖ 1 (15 oz.) can of chickpeas, drained and rinsed
- ❖ 2 tablespoons of olive oil.
- ❖ 1 teaspoon of garlic powder.
- ❖ 1 teaspoon of paprika.
- ❖ Add salt and pepper to taste.

## Instructions:
- Preheat the oven to 425° Fahrenheit (220° Celsius).
- Pat the chickpeas dry with a towel before spreading them on a baking sheet.
- Toss with olive oil, garlic powder, paprika, salt, and pepper until evenly coated.
- Roast for 25-30 minutes, until brown and crispy.

**Nutrition Facts:**
Each serving contains approximately 6g of protein.

**Modifications/Substitutes:**
For a variety of flavors, try adding spices such as cumin or chili powder.

# Edamame pods.

**Prep time: 5 minutes, Cook time: 5 minutes and Serving size: two cups.**

## Ingredients:
- ❖ 2 cups of edamame pods, fresh or frozen.
- ❖ Salt to taste.

## Instructions:
- In a pot, bring the water to a boil before adding the edamame pods.
- Cook for about 5 minutes, until tender.

- Drain and season with salt before serving.

**Nutrition facts:**
Each serving contains approximately 17g of protein.

**Modifications/Substitutes:**
Add garlic powder or chili flakes for added flavor.

## Cheese and Cracker Platter

**Prep time: 10 minutes, Cooking Time: None and Serving Size: Four servings**

### Ingredients:
- ❖ 8 oz cheese (cheddar, gouda, or your preference)
- ❖ 1 box of whole grain crackers.
- ❖ Optional: sliced fruits and nuts.

### Instructions:
- Slice the cheese into bite-sized pieces.
- Arrange the cheese and crackers on a dish.
- To add variation, mix it with some fruits or nuts.

**Nutrition Facts:**
Each serving contains approximately 8g of protein.

**Modification:**
For a lighter option, substitute low-fat cheese.

## Hummus with Vegetable Sticks

**Prep time: 10 minutes, Cooking Time: None and Serving Size: Four servings**

### Ingredients:
- ❖ 1 cup of hummus, either store-bought or homemade
- ❖ Assorted vegetable sticks (carrots, celery, and bell peppers)

**Instructions:**
- Arrange the vegetable sticks on a dish.
- Serve hummus in the center for dipping.

**Nutrition Facts:**
Each serving of hummus contains approximately 5g of protein.

**Modifications:**
For more taste, add spices like paprika to hummus.

# Almond Butter Energy Balls.

**Prep time: 15 minutes, Cooking Time: None and Serving size: twelve balls.**

## Ingredients:
- ❖ 1 cup rolled oats.
- ❖ 1/2 cup almond butter.
- ❖ 1/4 cup honey.
- ❖ Optional: dried fruit or chocolate chips.

## Instructions:
- In a bowl, combine the oats, almond butter, honey, and optional additions.
- Roll the mixture into tiny balls.
- Refrigerate for a minimum of 30 minutes before serving.
- Nutrition Facts: Each ball contains around 4g of protein.
- Modifications: If preferred, use peanut butter for almond butter.

# Greek Yogurt Dip and Pita Chips

**Prep time: 10 minutes, Cooking Time: None And Serving Size: Four servings**

## Ingredients:
- ❖ One cup plain Greek yogurt.
- ❖ 1 tablespoon of lemon juice.
- ❖ 1 teaspoon of garlic powder.
- ❖ Add salt and pepper to taste.
- ❖ 4 whole wheat pita bread, sliced into triangles.

**Instructions:**

- In a mixing bowl, combine Greek yogurt, lemon juice, garlic powder, salt, and pepper until smooth.
- Serve the dip with pita chips on the side.

**Nutrition Facts:**
Each serving contains approximately 10g of protein.

**Modifications:**
For added flavor, add herbs like dill or parsley

# Nut mixture (almonds, walnuts, etc.)

**Prep time: 5 minutes, Cooking Time: None and Serving Size: Four servings**

**Ingredients:**

- ❖ 1 cup mixed nuts (almonds, walnuts, cashews, and Brazil nuts).
- ❖ Optional: 1/4 teaspoon cinnamon or sea salt for taste.

**Instructions:**
Put all of the nuts in a bowl.
Sprinkle with salt or cinnamon if preferred.

**Nutrition facts:**
Each serving contains approximately 15g of protein.

**Modifications:**
Use unsalted nuts for a healthier alternative.

# Mini Caprese Skewers.

**Prep time: 10 minutes, Cooking Time: None and Serving Size: Four servings**

**Ingredients:**

- ❖ Twelve cherry tomatoes.
- ❖ Twelve tiny mozzarella balls.
- ❖ Fresh basil leaves.

- ❖ Balsamic glaze (to drizzle)
- ❖ Add salt and pepper to taste.

## Instructions:

- Thread cherry tomatoes, basil leaves, and mozzarella balls onto small skewers.
- Repeat until all ingredients have been utilized.
- Drizzle with balsamic glaze, then season with salt and pepper.

**Nutrition Facts:**

Each serving contains approximately 7g of protein.

**Modifications/Substitutes:**

For a dairy-free version, substitute vegan cheese.

## Cucumber Slices with Tuna Salad

Prep time: 10 minutes, Cooking Time: None and Serving Size: Four servings

## Ingredients:

- ❖ 1 canned tuna (5 oz.), drained
- ❖ 2 tablespoons of Greek yogurt or mayonnaise.
- ❖ 1 tbsp mustard.
- ❖ Add salt and pepper to taste.
- ❖ 1 cucumber sliced into rounds.

## Instructions:

- In a mixing bowl, combine tuna, Greek yogurt or mayonnaise, mustard, salt, and pepper.
- Top each cucumber slice with a scoop of tuna salad.

**Nutrition facts:**

Each serving contains approximately 15g of protein.

**Modifications/Substitutes:**

For added crunch, mix in diced celery or onion.

# Baked Sweet Potato Fries.

**Prep time: 10 minutes, Cook time: 25 minutes and Serving Size: Four servings**

## Ingredients:

- ❖ Two medium sweet potatoes, sliced into fries.
- ❖ 2 tablespoons of olive oil.
- ❖ Add salt and pepper to taste.
- ❖ Optional seasonings include paprika or garlic powder.

## Instructions:

- Preheat the oven to 425° Fahrenheit (220° Celsius).
- Toss sweet potato fries with olive oil, salt, pepper, and any spices.
- Spread on a baking sheet and bake for 25 minutes, until crispy.

**Nutrition Facts:**
Each serving contains approximately 4g of protein.

**Modifications:**
If you want, use normal potatoes.

# Chapter 8: Weekly Shopping list,  Meal Prep and Planning for Busy Days.



**Monday**
Breakfast: Steak and Eggs
Lunch: Hearty Salad with Grilled Chicken
Dinner: Roasted Lamb
Snack: Jerky (beef or turkey) and Greek Yogurt Dip with Pita Chips

**Tuesday**
Breakfast: Greek Yogurt Parfait with Nuts
Lunch: Tuna Salad in Lettuce Wraps
Dinner: Chicken Thighs with Garlic and Lemon
Snack: HardBoiled Eggs and Nut Mixture (almonds, walnuts)

**Wednesday**
Breakfast: Protein Overnight Oats
Lunch: Lentil Soup with Ham
Dinner: BBQ Brisket
Snack: Hummus with Vegetable Sticks

**Thursday**
Breakfast: Peanut Butter Banana Smoothie
Lunch: Turkey and Spinach Wraps
Dinner: Thai Red Curry Chicken
Snack: Chia Seed Pudding

**Friday**
Breakfast: Egg Muffins with Vegetables and Cheese
Lunch: Quinoa Salad with Chickpeas
Dinner: Stuffed Portobello Mushrooms with Sausage
Snack: Roasted Chickpeas and Cheese and Cracker Platter

**Saturday**
Breakfast: High Protein Pancakes
Lunch: Egg Salad with Wholc Grain Bread
Dinner: HerbCrusted Salmon Filets
Snack: Greek Yogurt Dip with Pita Chips

**Sunday**
Breakfast: Chia Seed Pudding with Berries
Lunch: Beef and Broccoli StirFry
Dinner: Classic Meatloaf with Mashed Potatoes
Snack: Nut Mixture (almonds, walnuts) and HardBoiled Eggs

## Week 1 Shopping List from Monday to Sunday

# Proteins

Steak, Lamb, Chicken, Ham, Ground Beef or Brisket, Eggs, Greek Yogurt, Cheese, Jerky, Sausage, Smoked Salmon, Shrimp, Ground Turkey

## Grains & Legumes

Whole Grain Bread, Quinoa, Chickpeas, Lentils, Pita Chips

## Vegetables

Mixed Salad Greens, Spinach, Broccoli, Bell Peppers, Portobello Mushrooms, Potatoes, Avocados, Garlic, Lemon, Cucumber, Sweet Potatoes

## Fruits

Bananas, Berries

## Other Essentials

Nuts (almonds, walnuts), Chia Seeds, Almond Butter, Hummus, Tahini Sauce, Bone Broth, Edamame Pods, Olive Oil, Vinegar

## Week 2: Daily Meal Plan from Monday to Sunday

**Monday**
Breakfast: Cottage Cheese, Fruit, and Honey
Lunch: Chicken Caesar Salad
Dinner: StirFried Tofu with Vegetables
Snack: Bone Broth and Hummus with Vegetable Sticks

**Tuesday**
Breakfast: Savory Oatmeal with a Poached Egg
Lunch: Mediterranean Chickpea Bowl

Dinner: Grilled Shrimp Skewers with Vegetables
Snack: Roasted Chickpeas

**Wednesday**
Breakfast: Protein Overnight Oats
Lunch: Beef and Broccoli StirFry
Dinner: BBQ Pulled Pork Sandwiches
Snack: Cheese and Cracker Platter

**Thursday**
Breakfast: Peanut Butter Banana Smoothie
Lunch: Falafel Wraps with Tahini Sauce
Dinner: Classic Meatloaf with Mashed Potatoes
Snack: Mini Caprese Skewers

**Friday**
Breakfast: High Protein Pancakes
Lunch: Tuna Salad in Lettuce Wraps
Dinner: Thai Red Curry Chicken
Snack: HardBoiled Eggs and Nut Mixture

**Saturday**
Breakfast: Egg Muffins with Vegetables and Cheese
Lunch: Stuffed Peppers with Ground Turkey
Dinner: HerbCrusted Salmon Filets
Snack: Greek Yogurt Dip with Pita Chips

**Sunday**
Breakfast: Chia Seed Pudding with Berries
Lunch: Quinoa Salad with Chickpeas
Dinner: Ratatouille with Grilled Sausages
Snack: Edamame Pods

## Week 2 Shopping List from Monday to Sunday

## Proteins

Chicken, Tofu, Ground Beef, Shrimp, Pork, Eggs, Greek Yogurt, Cheese, Sausages

## Grains & Legumes

Whole Grain Bread, Quinoa, Chickpeas, Lentils, Pita Chips

## Vegetables

Mixed Salad Greens, Spinach, Broccoli, Bell Peppers, Portobello Mushrooms, Avocados, Garlic, Lemon, Cucumber, Sweet Potatoes, Cauliflower, Zucchini

**Fruits**

Bananas, Berries

## Other Essentials

Nuts (almonds, walnuts), Chia Seeds, Almond Butter, Hummus, Tahini Sauce, Bone Broth, Edamame Pods, Olive Oil, Vinegar, Caprese ingredients

## Week 3: Daily Meal Plan from Monday to Sunday

**Monday**
Breakfast: Morning Sausages
Lunch: Grilled Chicken with Quinoa Bowl
Dinner: HerbCrusted Salmon Filets
Snack: Nut Mixture and HardBoiled Eggs

**Tuesday**
Breakfast: Greek Yogurt Parfait with Nuts
Lunch: Tuna Salad Lettuce Wraps
Dinner: StirFried Tofu with Vegetables
Snack: Almond Butter Energy Balls

**Wednesday**
Breakfast: Quinoa Breakfast Bowl with Almonds
Lunch: Lentil Soup with Ham
Dinner: BBQ Brisket
Snack: Hummus with Vegetable Sticks

**Thursday**
Breakfast: High Protein Pancakes
Lunch: Egg Salad with Whole Grain Bread
Dinner: Classic Meatloaf with Mashed Potatoes
Snack: Roasted Chickpeas

**Friday**
Breakfast: Chia Seed Pudding with Berries
Lunch: Mediterranean Chickpea Bowl
Dinner: Thai Red Curry Chicken
Snack: Cheese and Cracker Platter

**Saturday**
Breakfast: Savory Oatmeal with a Poached Egg
Lunch: Beef and Broccoli StirFry
Dinner: Stuffed Portobello Mushrooms with Sausage
Snack: Greek Yogurt Dip with Pita Chips

**Sunday**
Breakfast: Protein Overnight Oats
Lunch: Stuffed Peppers with Ground Turkey
Dinner: Ratatouille with Grilled Sausages
Snack: Mini Caprese Skewers

## Week 3 Shopping List from Monday to Sunday

## Proteins

Chicken, Sausages, Tofu, Ground Beef, Eggs, Greek Yogurt, Cheese, Pork

## Grains & Legumes

Whole Grain Bread, Quinoa, Chickpeas, Lentils, Pita Chips

## Vegetables

Mixed Salad Greens, Spinach, Broccoli, Bell Peppers, Portobello Mushrooms, Avocados, Garlic, Lemon, Cucumber, Sweet Potatoes, Cauliflower, Zucchini

## Fruits

Bananas, Berries

## Other Essentials

Nuts (almonds, walnuts), Chia Seeds, Almond Butter, Hummus, Tahini Sauce, Bone Broth, Edamame Pods, Olive Oil, Vinegar

**Monday**
Breakfast: Steak and Eggs
Lunch: Grilled Chicken with Quinoa Bowl
Dinner: Roasted Lamb
Snack: Jerky and Greek Yogurt Dip with Pita Chips

**Tuesday**
Breakfast: Cottage Cheese, Fruit, and Honey
Lunch: Chicken Caesar Salad
Dinner: StirFried Tofu with Vegetables
Snack: Almond Butter Energy Balls

**Wednesday**
Breakfast: Protein Overnight Oats
Lunch: Tuna Salad Lettuce Wraps
Dinner: BBQ Brisket
Snack: Hummus with Vegetable Sticks

**Thursday**
Breakfast: Savory Oatmeal with a Poached Egg
Lunch: Mediterranean Chickpea Bowl
Dinner: Classic Meatloaf with Mashed Potatoes
Snack: Mini Caprese Skewers

**Friday**
Breakfast: Peanut Butter Banana Smoothie
Lunch: Turkey and Spinach Wraps
Dinner: Thai Red Curry Chicken
Snack: Roasted Chickpeas

**Saturday**
Breakfast: High Protein Pancakes
Lunch: Quinoa Salad with Chickpeas
Dinner: Stuffed Portobello Mushrooms with Sausage
Snack: Cheese and Cracker Platter

**Sunday**
Breakfast: Chia Seed Pudding with Berries
Lunch: Egg Salad with Whole Grain Bread

Dinner: HerbCrusted Salmon Filets
Snack: Nut Mixture and HardBoiled Eggs

## Week 4 Shopping List from Monday to Sunday

## Proteins

Steak, Chicken, Ground Beef, Sausages, Tofu, Eggs, Greek Yogurt, Cheese, Pork

## Grains & Legumes

Whole Grain Bread, Quinoa

**Make-ahead dishes, freezer-friendly alternatives, and batch-cooking techniques are to help you streamline your meal preparation.**

Here are some excellent make-ahead recipes, freezer-friendly alternatives, and batch-cooking techniques to help you streamline your meal preparation:

## Make-ahead recipes

### Balsamic-glazed mini meatloaves

Prepare small meatloaves ahead of time and refrigerate them for up to three days. They can also be frozen for long-term storage.

### Vegetarian Antipasto Salad

Marinate all ingredients except the greens in advance. For a refreshing salad, toss everything together right before serving.

### Lasagna with Meat Sauce

Prepare the lasagna ahead of time and refrigerate overnight. Bake the following day or freeze for later.

### Creamy Chicken Pot Pies

Assemble the pot pies and freeze them completely. When the necessity arises, bake directly from the freezer.

### Quick White Beans and Sausage Stew

This stew can be cooked ahead of time and refrigerated or frozen. It reheats nicely.

**Mason Jar Instant Noodle Soup**
Layer all of the ingredients in a jar, refrigerate, and then add hot water when ready to serve.

**Chicken Curry**
Cook a large quantity of chicken curry and freeze it for easy dinners later.

**Freezer-Friendly Options**
**Roasted Eggplant Veggie Burgers**
These burgers can be cooked in bulk and frozen individually for convenient meals.

**Quiche Lorraine**
Prepare the quiche ahead of time; it may be kept in the refrigerator for a few days or frozen for months.

**Slow Cooker Chicken Pozole Verde**
Make a large amount and freeze the leftovers for future meals.

**Savory oatmeal with a poached egg.**
While oatmeal is best eaten fresh, you can make individual servings and reheat them quickly.

**Peanut Butter Banana Smoothie Packs**
Pre-portion the ingredients into bags and freeze them. When you're ready to eat, blend with milk or yogurt.

**Batch Cooking Tips**
Plan your meals:
Create a weekly or monthly meal plan that includes batch cookable recipes.

**Cook in batches.**
Prepare huge quantities of recipes such as soups, stews, and casseroles that may be divided across numerous meals.

**Use freezer-friendly containers.**

Invest in excellent freezer-safe containers to prevent freezer burn.

**Label everything.**

Label containers with names and dates so you know what you have and when it was manufactured.

**Cook once and eat twice:**

Make extra dishes of dinner that can be used as lunch the following day.

**Utilize Your Slow Cooker**:

Slow cookers are ideal for preparing huge quantities of food with minimal effort.

**Preparing Ingredients ahead of time:**

Cut veggies, marinade proteins, or cook grains ahead of time to make dinner preparation is easier during the week. Include basic recommendations for developing a weekly schedule that promotes simple, meat-based meals with minimal daily preparation.

**Quick tips for a weekly routine.**

**Plan Your Meal Ahead:**

Set aside time each week (such as Sunday) to plan your meals. Casseroles, soups, and stews are examples of meals that may be prepared ahead of time and kept for the week.

**Batch Cook Proteins:**

Cook greater servings of protein, such as chicken, beef, or turkey, at once. Grill or bake several pieces and keep them in the fridge for easy access all week.

**Use versatile ingredients.**

Choose foods that can be utilized in several meals. Grilled chicken, for example, can be incorporated into salads, wraps, or served alongside rice.

**Preparing Ingredients in Advance:**
Prepare vegetables and marinade meat ahead of time. Keep them in containers so they're ready to cook when you need them.

**Use Freezer-Friendly Meals:**
Prepare and freeze dishes such as meatballs, casseroles, and chili. This provides you with ready-to-eat options on hectic days.

**Keep it simple.**
Choose dishes that have fewer ingredients or require less cooking time. One-pan meals or sheet pan dinners can help you save time cleaning up.

**Incorporate leftovers:**
Plan meals that allow for imaginative use of leftovers. For example, roast a chicken on Sunday and use the leftovers in sandwiches or salads throughout the week.

**Create a Cooking Schedule:**
Designate specific days for food preparation. For example, cook proteins on Sunday, prepare sides on Wednesday, and put together quick dinners on Friday.

**Use slow cookers or instant pots.**
These appliances let you set it and forget it. Prepare stews or meats in the morning and arrive home for a meal.

**Use canned or frozen options.**
Stock up on canned beans, frozen vegetables, and pre-cooked grains to easily add protein and fiber to your meals with minimal preparation.

# Chapter 9: Overcoming Common Challenges

Maintaining a high-protein diet can be difficult for a variety of reasons, including managing carb cravings, remaining on track when eating out, and regulating the expenses of quality meat. Here's how to deal with these typical concerns effectively.

- **Handling Cravings for Carbs**
  Cravings for carbohydrates can disrupt your diet plans. Here are some techniques for overcoming them.
- Balanced meals: Ensure that each meal has an appropriate amount of protein, healthy fats, and fiber. This combo can help you stay full and lessen your cravings for carbohydrates. For example, serve grilled chicken with quinoa and steamed broccoli.
- Healthy alternatives: Replace processed carbohydrates with more nutritious options such as whole grains, legumes, or starchy vegetables. For example, rather than white rice or bread, choose quinoa or sweet potatoes. Consider cauliflower rice as a low-carb option.
- Stay Hydrated: Thirst might be mistaken for hunger. Drink plenty of water throughout the day to help reduce cravings. Herbal teas can also help you keep hydrated while providing a soothing alternative.
- Mindful eating: Mindful eating entails paying attention to your hunger signs and eating slowly. This can help you tell when you're actually hungry and when you're desiring comfort foods. To slow down your eating pace, try putting your fork down between each bite.
- Snack smartly. Keep protein-rich snacks on hand, such as Greek yogurt, almonds, or hard-boiled eggs. These can help satiate hunger without relying on carbohydrate-laden foods.
- Plan your indulgences: Allow yourself the odd treat in moderation. Planning a little dessert or a favorite carb-rich meal on occasion will help reduce feelings of deprivation, which can contribute to binge eating.
- **Staying on Track While Eating Out**
  Eating out might be difficult when trying to follow a high-protein diet. Here are some strategies for staying on track:

- Review menus ahead of time: Before going out, look up restaurant menus online. This helps you to locate protein-rich options and plan your order ahead of time. Many eateries now provide nutritional information online.
- Choose protein-rich dishes: Choose meals centered on lean proteins like grilled chicken, fish, or lentils. Salads with additional protein (such as chicken or beans) are also excellent options. Avoid fried or breaded alternatives, as they can add extra calories.
- Portion Control: Restaurants frequently serve greater portions than are necessary. To avoid overeating, consider splitting a dish or ordering a half serving. Alternatively, you might request a doggy bag at the beginning of the meal and portion out half your meal right away.
- Request Modifications: Do not be afraid to ask for changes, such as dressing on the side or replacing fries with a side salad. Most restaurants accommodate dietary restrictions.
- Skip the bread basket. Politely decline the bread basket and any complimentary carb-heavy beginnings, which may lead to overeating before your dinner arrives.
- Focus on the sides: Choose sides that compliment your protein and add nutritious value, such as steamed vegetables or a side salad, rather than starchy sides like mashed potatoes or rice.
- **Managing the Cost of Quality Meat.**
  Quality meat can be costly, however there are useful cost-management strategies:
  Buy in bulk. Purchasing larger quantities of beef can result in significant savings. Consider purchasing family packs and freezing them for later use. Look into local farms or butcher businesses that may provide bulk purchase at a discount.
- Plan your meals: Create a weekly meal plan that integrates meat strategically. This helps to reduce waste and ensures you use what you buy. Use leftover meat in salads, wraps, or stir-fries later in the week.
- Consider Alternative Cuts: Less popular pieces of meat are frequently less expensive, but can be just as tasty when prepared correctly. Consider using chicken thighs instead of breasts or chuck roast instead of ribeye. Slow simmering harder cuts can turn them soft and tasty.

- Utilize Sales & Discounts: Keep an eye on the sales at your local grocery shop and stock up when quality meats are reduced. Joining loyalty programs can result in further discounts.
  Consider plant-based proteins. Include plant-based proteins such as beans, lentils, and tofu in your diet alongside meat-based meals. They are frequently less priced and offer superior nutrients.
- Meal prep with leftovers: Cook larger dinners with meat so that leftovers may be used in imaginative ways throughout the week, such as turning roasted chicken into chicken salad or tacos.

- **Managing Social Pressures**
  Social interactions can make it tough to stick to your nutritional goals.
- Communicate your goals: Inform your friends and family about your dietary choices so that they can support you at social gatherings or dinners out.
  Bring your own dish. Bring a high-protein dish that corresponds with your dietary objectives to potlucks or events to ensure you have something healthy to eat.
- Practice Saying No: It is acceptable to decline food offerings that do not correspond with your goals without feeling bad. You can respectfully decline dessert or additional portions by stating that you are full or saving room for something else later.

- **Emotional Eating Emotional triggers can contribute to unhealthy eating behaviors**.
  - Identify triggers: Keep a journal to track when you have cravings triggered by emotions rather than hunger. Recognizing these patterns is the first step toward addressing them.
  - Find alternatives: Instead of turning to food during stressful times, try better coping techniques like going for a walk, practicing yoga, meditating, or indulging in mind-stimulating hobbies.
  - Stay accountable: Share your goals with someone who can hold you accountable during difficult times, such as a friend, family member, or a nutrition and health support group.

**Practical advice and solutions for dealing with these issues, such as snack options, substitute suggestions, and cost-effective recipes.**

Here are practical recommendations and solutions for dealing with typical obstacles when following a high-protein diet, such as snack options, substitute ideas, and cost-effective dishes.

## 1. Managing Cravings for Carbs

- Healthy Snack Options:
  Greek Yogurt with Berries: A high-protein snack that quenches sweet cravings.
- Nut Butter with Apple Slices: Provides healthy fats and protein while satiating hunger.
- Hummus with Veggies: This hearty dip goes great with crisp veggies like carrots and cucumbers.

**Consider using quinoa or cauliflower rice as a low-carb substitute for white rice.**

**Replace standard pasta with zucchini noodles or whole-grain choices to boost fiber and protein.**

## 2. Budget-Friendly Recipes

- Veggie Protein Chili: Made with canned beans, tomatoes, and seasonings, this dish is both hearty and affordable.
- Spicy Cajun Chicken Quinoa: A simple dish made with chicken thighs, quinoa, and spices that can be prepared in bulk.

## 3. Keeping on Track While Eating Out

- To find protein-rich selections on restaurant menus, check online.
- To make meals healthy, choose grilled or baked proteins over fried choices.
- Pack high-protein snacks such as beef jerky, protein bars, or hard-boiled eggs to avoid impulsive carb-heavy selections during long trips.

**Substitution suggestion: Request whole grain bread instead of white for sandwiches. Request extra vegetables instead of fries or chips as a side.**

**4. Cost Management for Quality Meat: Budget-Friendly Protein Sources.**

- Canned Fish: Tuna and salmon are low-cost protein options for salads and sandwiches.
- Eggs are a versatile and economical ingredient that may be used in a variety of meals ranging from breakfast to dinner.
- Lentils and beans: These legumes are not only inexpensive, but also high in protein. Use them in soups, stews, and salads.

**Cook huge batches of food, such as Mexican Chicken Stew with Quinoa & Beans or Vegan Chickpea Curry, to preserve for numerous days.**
**Make a large quantity of lentil soup or chili; it freezes well and reheats easily.**

**5. Inexpensive Recipe Ideas:**

- Pumpkin Protein Pancakes: Combine canned pumpkin with oats to make a nutritious and inexpensive breakfast alternative.
- Sheet Pan Chicken Fajitas: Quick to make with few ingredients; chicken thighs are frequently less expensive than breasts.

## Additional practical solutions.

- **Meal Preparation Strategies:**
  Set some time each week to prepare meals in advance. Cook proteins in bulk, such as chicken thighs or ground beef, and divide them into portions for convenient access throughout the week.
- Use freezer-friendly containers to store foods like chili or casseroles for easy reheating on busy days.
- Creative Leftover Ideas: Use leftover grilled chicken in a salad or wrap for lunch.
- Extra cooked quinoa can be added to breakfast bowls with eggs or blended into vegetable stir-fries.

- Stock your cupboard with staples such as canned beans, lentils, rice, quinoa, and pasta. These can be used as the foundation for a variety of high-protein meals while remaining affordable.

## Strategies for navigating exceptional situations such as social gatherings or travel while adhering to a meat-first diet.

Here are some tips for dealing with exceptional events, such as social gatherings or travel, while sticking to a meat-first diet. These pointers can help you handle diverse settings without jeopardizing your nutritional goals.

### Managing Social Gatherings

### Plan ahead:

If you know you'll be attending a gathering, have a protein-rich snack before you go. This can help lessen hunger and the temptation to eat carb-heavy appetizers.

### Bring your own dish.

Offer to bring a protein-rich food that is appropriate for your diet, such as a meat and cheese platter, grilled chicken skewers, or a robust salad with protein. This ensures that you have something to appreciate.

### Choose Wisely.

On occasion, choose protein-rich alternatives. Look for options such as grilled meats, seafood, and cheese platters. Avoid breaded or fried foods that are high in carbohydrates.

### Portion Control

For non-protein products, choose smaller servings. Use a smaller plate whenever possible to help reduce serving sizes.

- Drink water or zero-calorie beverages to stay hydrated and reduce cravings for snacks and desserts.
- When ordering, request sauces or dressings on the side to limit your intake.

**Additional Tips:**

- Mindful Eating: Pay attention to hunger cues and eat gently so you can enjoy your food without overeating.
- Set Realistic Goals: Allow for some flexibility at social gatherings or trips without feeling bad; moderation is essential.
- Stay Prepared: Always bring a backup plan for meals and snacks in case possibilities are restricted at your destination.

# Chapter 10: Tracking Progress and Maintaining Results

Monitoring your progress on a high-protein diet is critical to reaching your health and fitness objectives. This chapter will teach you how to track changes in energy levels, body composition, and mental clarity to keep you motivated and on track.

## Monitoring Energy Levels.

Keep a food diary to track what you eat and how you feel throughout the day. Take note of any changes in energy, mood, or hunger. MyNetDiary and other apps make it simple to track your food consumption and energy levels 1.

- **Assess Physical Performance:** Consider how your energy levels affect your workouts. Can you lift heavier weights or do more reps? Improved performance frequently signals improved energy management.
- **Identify Patterns:** Look for similarities between what you consume and how you feel. If certain meals give you more energy while others make you tired, change your diet accordingly.

## Tracking Body Composition

- **Regular Measurements:** Measure your waist, hips, and other important areas every few weeks. This can assist you identify changes in body composition that may not be reflected on the scale.
- **Body Fat Percentage:** Consider utilizing body fat calipers or a smart scale to calculate body fat percentage. This offers a more complete picture of your progress than just weight loss.
- **Progress images:** Take images every several weeks with consistent lighting and settings. Visual comparisons can be motivational and allow you to notice changes that measurements may not detect.
- **Consult Professionals:** If feasible, work with a licensed nutritionist or personal trainer who can offer advice on how to successfully track body composition 3.

## Enhancing Mental Clarity

- Journal your cognitive performance throughout the day. Take note of any foods that appear to improve or impede cognitive performance.
- **Evaluate Protein Intake:** Make sure you're getting enough protein at each meal. Protein is essential for neurotransmitter function, which influences mood and mental acuity 4.
- Monitor your water intake because dehydration might impair cognitive function. Aim for at least 8 cups of water per day, or more depending on activity level.

## Sustainable Results

- **Set Realistic ambitions:** To stay motivated, break down enormous ambitions into smaller, more manageable benchmarks. To keep motivated about your development, celebrate tiny triumphs along the road.
- **Adjust as Needed:** As you progress, reassess your nutritional requirements and goals. Protein consumption may need to be adjusted depending on your exercise level or body composition objectives.
- **Stay Flexible:** Life is unpredictable; give yourself some leeway in your diet without guilt. The goal is to return to a high-protein diet following any indulgences or aberrations.
- **Community Support:** Participate in communities (online forums, local groups) with similar dietary goals. Sharing experiences and tips can boost motivation and accountability.

## Advice on changing the diet depending on results, including suggestions for fine-tuning quantities, protein intake, and meal scheduling.

Here are some helpful hints for fine-tuning quantities, protein consumption, and meal scheduling to keep you on track.

### Fine-Tuning Portions

- **Evaluate Your Plate:** Use the "plate method" to visualize portion sizes. Fill half of your plate with veggies, one-fourth with lean protein, and the remaining quarter with whole grains or starchy vegetables. This balance allows you to keep your calorie consumption under control while still getting enough nutrition.

- **Listen to Your Body:** Pay attention to hunger and fullness signals. If you're constantly hungry after meals, try increasing your portion sizes of protein and fiber-rich foods.
- **Use Measuring Tools:** Begin by using measuring cups or a food scale to better comprehend portion sizes. Over time, you'll develop a visual sense of acceptable portion sizes without having to measure each meal.

**Adjusting Protein Intake**

- **Calculate Your Needs:** Aim for 1.2 to 2.0 grams of protein per kilogram of body weight, depending on your activity level and goals (e.g., weight loss, muscle gain). 13. Adjust this range based on your body's response.
- **Protein Distribution:** Spread your protein consumption throughout the day by incorporating a protein source into each meal and snack. Aim for 15-30 g of protein every meal 3. This can aid to preserve muscle mass and increase satiety.

Include a diverse range of protein sources, such as lean meats, fish, eggs, dairy, legumes, and plant-based proteins. This guarantees that you obtain all of the necessary amino acids while keeping meals exciting.

**Optimizing Meal Timing**

- **Prioritize Protein at Breakfast:** Begin your day with a high-protein breakfast to help control your hunger throughout the day 3. Greek yogurt with fruit or an egg-based dish can help boost your metabolism.
- **Pre- and Post-Workout Nutrition:** If you exercise frequently, eat a protein-rich snack or meal before and after each workout to aid in recuperation and muscle growth. A protein drink with a banana or a turkey sandwich are good examples of protein-carbohydrate combinations.

- **Plan Meals Around Activity Levels:** On days with more activity, slightly increase your carbohydrate consumption around workouts while keeping optimal protein levels. On rest days, focus on protein and healthy fats.

## Budget-Friendly Protein Strategies

- **Choose Affordable Proteins:** Include low-cost protein sources such as ground beef, canned fish (tuna or salmon), lentils, beans, eggs, and chicken thighs 4. These options offer great nutrition without breaking the pocketbook.
- **Batch Cooking:** Make huge batches of freezer-friendly foods like chili or lentil soup. This saves time and money while ensuring that you have nutritious meals available as needed.
- **Use Leftovers Creatively:** Repurpose leftovers to create new meals. For example, leftover grilled chicken can be used in salads or wraps for lunch the following day.

## Additional Tools.

- **Diet journals:** Consider keeping a physical diet journal or planner to physically record your meals, snacks, and feelings throughout the day. This can help you be more attentive about your eating habits.
- **Wearable fitness trackers:**
- Devices such as Fitbit and Apple Watch can help you track your activity levels as well as your dietary consumption. Many of these gadgets integrate with nutrition apps to provide full tracking.

## Tips to Stay Consistent

- **create Specific Goals:** Determine what you want to accomplish (e.g., weight loss, muscle gain) and utilize your preferred app to create specific targets.
  Schedule weekly or biweekly check-ins to assess your progress in the app. Adjust your goals as appropriate based on the information you get.

- **Engage with Communities:** Many apps have community forums or groups. Engaging with people might help you stay motivated and supported during your journey.

# Chapter 11: Advanced Nutrition for High Performers.

Nutrition is critical for athletes and other people who are physically active in terms of performance, recovery, and overall health. This chapter discusses meal scheduling around workouts and includes recovery-focused recipes to help you optimize your nutrition for peak performance.

## Meal Timing for Workout

### Pre-workout Nutrition

- **Timing:** Aim to eat a balanced lunch with carbs and protein 3-4 hours before your workout. If you're getting closer to your workout (1-2 hours), choose a lighter, easier-to-digest food.

**What to eat?**

- 3-4 hours before: A complete dinner, such as grilled chicken with quinoa and vegetables.

   **1-2 hours before:** Snack on Greek yogurt with honey and berries or a peanut butter banana sandwich.8

## Quick Digesting Options (30 Minutes Ahead):

A half banana or a cup of applesauce.
A little protein smoothie or a serving of pretzels.

## Post-workout Nutrition

- **Timing:** Eat a meal or snack within 60 minutes of exercising to restore glycogen levels and aid in muscle recovery.

**What to eat?**

- **Post-Workout Meal:** A recovery smoothie with low-fat milk, protein powder, and fruit, or turkey on a whole-grain wrap with vegetables.

Quick options include low-fat chocolate milk and low-fat yogurt with oats.

Macronutrient Ratio: For optimal energy replenishment and muscle regeneration, aim for a post-workout meal with a carbohydrate-to-protein ratio of roughly 3:1.

## Recovery-Oriented Recipes

### Recovery Smoothie

**Ingredients:**
- ❖ 1 cup almond milk (or low-fat milk)
- ❖ 1 scoop protein powder (plant-based or whey)
- ❖ 1 banana.
- ❖ 1/2 cup spinach (optional).
- ❖ 1 tablespoon of peanut butter.

**Instructions:**
- Combine all ingredients and blend until smooth.
- Serve shortly following your workout to maximize healing.

**Nutritional Benefits:**
This smoothie has quick-digesting carbohydrates from the banana, protein for muscle repair, and healthy fats from the peanut butter.

### Turkey and Quinoa Bowl

**Ingredients:**
- ❖ 1 cup cooked quinoa.
- ❖ 4 ounces ground turkey (cooked).
- ❖ 1/2 cup steaming broccoli.
- ❖ 1/4 avocado, sliced
- ❖ Drizzle with olive oil and lemon juice

**Instructions:**

- In a bowl, combine cooked quinoa, ground turkey, and steamed broccoli.
- Top with avocado slices, drizzle with olive oil, and squeeze lemon juice over top.

**Nutritional Benefits:**

This bowl is packed in protein from turkey and quinoa and contains healthy fats from avocado, making it ideal for post-workout recovery.

## Sweet potato and black bean tacos.

## Ingredients:

- ❖ Two small sweet potatoes, chopped
- ❖ One can of black beans, rinsed and drained
- ❖ Corn tortillas
- ❖ Salsa or Pico de Gallo
- ❖ Fresh cilantro (optional).

## Instructions:

Roast chopped sweet potatoes at 400°F (200°C) for about 25 minutes, or until tender.

## Warm the corn tortillas in a skillet.

Make tacos with roasted sweet potatoes, black beans, salsa, and cilantro.

Sweet potatoes give complex carbohydrates for long-term energy, while black beans contribute protein and fiber.

## Additional Tips for High Performers:

- **Hydration is essential:** Stay hydrated before, during, and after your workouts. Drink plenty of water throughout the day, and consider electrolyte drinks for longer or more severe workouts.
- **Experiment During Training:** Use training sessions to experiment with different diets and timings to determine what works best for your body before competition.
- **Listen to Your Body:** Be aware of how different foods affect your performance and recovery. To achieve the best outcomes, adjust your diet depending on personal experiences.

Set specific performance goals for your nutrition plan (such as increasing endurance or strength) and alter your intake as you advance.

## Increased protein requirements for muscle growth and endurance.

Athletes and highly active people have special dietary needs, notably in terms of protein intake. Understanding these requirements is critical for achieving peak performance, recuperation, and muscular growth.

## Protein requirements

- **Muscle Gain:** Athletes who train to build muscle often require additional protein to promote muscle repair and growth. The daily protein intake recommendation is 1.2 to 2.0 grams per kilogram of body weight (about 0.55 to 0.9 grams per pound). This greater consumption promotes muscle protein synthesis following resistance training.

**Endurance Training:** Endurance athletes require protein, but their major focus should be on carbs to provide sustained energy. They typically require approximately 1.2 to 1.4 grams of protein per kilogram of body weight. Adequate protein aids in recovery and muscle maintenance, although it is secondary to carbohydrate requirements for energy.

## Specific Guidelines for High-Performance Diets

Meal Timing

Pre-workout Nutrition:

Aim to eat a balanced lunch that includes carbohydrates and protein 3-4 hours before your activity. If you're getting closer to your workout (1-2 hours), choose a lighter, easier-to-digest food.

Examples include:

Full Meal: Grilled chicken, quinoa, and vegetables.

Snack options include Greek yogurt with honey or a banana with nut butter.

## Post-workout Nutrition:

Consume a meal or snack within 30-60 minutes of training to restore glycogen stores and aid in muscle regeneration.
Concentrate on a combination of protein and carbohydrates.
Post-Workout Meal: A smoothie with low-fat milk, protein powder, and fruit, or a turkey sandwich on whole-grain bread.
Quick options include low-fat chocolate milk or a protein snack.

## Macronutrient ratios.

To maximize performance, modify your macronutrient ratios based on your training intensity:
**Light training:** 1/4 carbs, 1/4 protein, and 1/2 fruits and vegetables.
**Moderate Training:** 1/3 carbs, 1/3 protein, and 1/3 fruits/vegetables.
**Hard Training:** 1/2 carbs, 1/4 protein, 1/4 vegetables, with fruit on the side.

## Recovery-Oriented Recipes

### Protein-Rich Recovery Smoothie

**Ingredients:**
- ❖ 1 cup low-fat milk.
- ❖ 1 scoop of protein powder.
- ❖ 1 banana.
- ❖ A handful of spinach (optional).

**Instructions:**
- Blend all ingredients until smooth, then eat shortly after your workout.

# Turkey Quinoa Bowl

**Ingredients:**

- ❖ 1 cup cooked quinoa.
- ❖ 4 ounces ground turkey (cooked).
- ❖ Steamed broccoli
- ❖ Avocado slices

**Instructions:**

- Place all of the ingredients in a bowl and sprinkle with olive oil.

# Sweet potato and black bean tacos.

**Ingredients:**

- ❖ Diced sweet potatoes, roasted
- ❖ Canned black beans (drained
- ❖ Corn tortillas

**Instructions:**

- Fill tortillas with sweet potatoes and black beans, then top with salsa.

# Additional Tips for High Performers:

- Stay hydrated before, during, and after workouts. Water is crucial for performance, and electrolyte drinks can help with prolonged activity.
- **Flexible Eating Plans:** Tailor your food intake to your workout schedule and energy needs. To increase energy levels, consider higher carbohydrate meals around workout times.
- **Listen to Your Body:** Track how different foods affect your performance and recuperation. To achieve the best outcomes, adjust your diet depending on personal experiences.

**Incorporating natural supplements into a meat-based diet can improve performance, recovery, and overall health, particularly for those seeking fitness.**

**Here are some important supplements to consider:**

### Collagen and Benefits:

Collagen is a protein that promotes joint health, skin elasticity, and muscle regeneration. It is especially good for athletes who put a strain on their joints during intensive exercise.

It may help reduce joint pain and increase flexibility, making it simpler to live an active lifestyle.

### How To Use:

Collagen powder can be ingested by mixing it into smoothies, coffee, or yogurt. Aim for roughly 10 grams per day for the best results.

### Electrolytes and Benefits:

Electrolytes (sodium, potassium, magnesium, and calcium) are essential for hydration and muscular function. They aid to prevent cramps and maintain fluid balance, especially after extended exercise.

Replenishing electrolytes after a workout can improve recovery and performance.

### How To Use:

Consider electrolyte powders or tablets, which can be mixed with water during or after exercise. Look for low-sugar products with a well-balanced electrolyte blend.

### Creatine and Benefits:

Creatine is a naturally occurring chemical present in meat that aids energy production during high-intensity exercise. It can boost strength, increase lean muscle mass, and speed up recovery.

Creatine supplementation has been shown in studies to increase muscular mass and strength significantly.

**How To Use:**

A normal dose is 3-5 grams per day, which can be taken before or after exercise. It is frequently advised to load with greater dosages (20 grams divided into four doses) for the first week before switching to the maintenance dose.

**Omega 3 Fatty Acids and Benefits:**

Omega-3s (found in fish oil) promote heart health, reduce inflammation, and may help with muscle recovery after exercise.
They are important fatty acids that support brain function and overall wellness.

**How To Use:**

Aim for 1-3 grams of combined EPA and DHA (the active forms of omega-3) per day via fish oil supplements or by eating fatty fish such as salmon or mackerel.

**Vitamin D and Benefits:**

Vitamin D is essential for bone health, immunity, and muscle performance. It also influences protein synthesis.
Many people have insufficient vitamin D levels, particularly those who spend little time outside.

## How To Use:

A daily dosage of 1000-2000 IU is often suggested, particularly during months with little sunshine exposure.

**Branched Chain Amino Acids (BCAAs) and Benefits:**

BCAAs (leucine, isoleucine, and valine) may minimize muscular soreness after exercises and may inhibit muscle breakdown while exercising.
When taken before or after a workout, they can help with recovery and growth.

**How To Use:**

A typical dose is 5-10 grams before or after an exercise, combined with water or your preferred beverage.

# Chapter 12: The Future of Your Primal Plate Lifestyle

Embracing a Primal Plate lifestyle is not just a dietary choice; it's a commitment to sustainable, health-focused eating that can lead to long-term wellness. To ensure that this lifestyle remains enjoyable and sustainable, consider the following strategies: seasonal eating, balanced variety, and mindful adjustments.

## 1. Seasonal Eating

- Embrace Local Produce: Eating seasonally means choosing fruits and vegetables that are in season in your area. This not only supports local farmers but also ensures that you're consuming fresh, nutrient-dense foods at their peak flavor and nutritional value.
- Plan Your Meals Around Seasons: Create meal plans that highlight seasonal ingredients. For example, enjoy hearty root vegetables in the fall and refreshing salads with summer produce. This approach keeps your meals exciting and varied throughout the year.
- Preserve Seasonal Foods: Consider canning, freezing, or fermenting seasonal produce to enjoy year-round. For instance, you can make tomato sauce in the summer and freeze it for use in winter meals.

## 2. Balanced Variety

- Incorporate Diverse Protein Sources: While a meat-based diet focuses heavily on animal proteins, it's important to include a variety of sources such as fish, poultry, eggs, and high-quality dairy. This ensures a broader spectrum of nutrients.
- Explore Different Cooking Methods: Experiment with grilling, roasting, braising, and slow cooking to prepare your meats and vegetables. Different methods can enhance flavors and textures, keeping meals interesting.
- Include Healthy Fats: Don't shy away from healthy fats like olive oil, avocados, nuts, and seeds. These not only add flavor but also provide essential fatty acids that support overall health.

### 3. Mindful Adjustments

- Listen to Your Body: Pay attention to how different foods make you feel. If certain foods cause discomfort or fatigue, consider adjusting your intake or eliminating them from your diet.
- Monitor Your Progress: Keep track of how your body responds to the Primal Plate lifestyle over time. Adjust your macronutrient ratios based on your activity levels and fitness goals. For example, if you're training for an endurance event, you may need to increase your carbohydrate intake slightly.
- Stay Flexible: Life is dynamic; allow yourself the flexibility to adapt your diet as needed. Whether it's accommodating social events or adjusting for seasonal changes in food availability, being adaptable helps maintain long-term adherence to your lifestyle.

## Embracing the Primal Plate Lifestyle: Adaptability and Long-Term Success

As you adopt the Primal Plate lifestyle, it's important to view this approach to eating as flexible and adaptable. This mindset will help you cultivate a sustainable relationship with food that supports your health and fitness goals over the long term.

### 1. Flexibility is Key

- Adapt to Your Needs: Life is full of changes—your schedule, activity levels, and even your taste preferences may shift over time. Embrace the flexibility of the Primal Plate lifestyle by adjusting your meals and snacks to fit your current needs. If you find yourself craving something different, don't hesitate to explore new recipes or ingredients that align with your principles.
- Occasional Indulgences: Allow yourself the freedom to enjoy occasional treats or meals that may not strictly adhere to your usual guidelines. Whether it's a slice of birthday cake or a favorite dish at a restaurant, these moments can enhance your overall enjoyment of food without derailing your progress. The key is moderation and mindfulness.

### 2. Room for Variety

- Experiment with New Foods: The Primal Plate lifestyle encourages exploration! Try incorporating new fruits, vegetables, and proteins into your meals. This not only keeps your diet interesting but also exposes you to a wider range of nutrients that can benefit your health.

- Culinary Creativity: Use cooking as an opportunity for creativity. Experiment with different herbs, spices, and cooking techniques to transform familiar ingredients into exciting new dishes. Join cooking classes or watch online tutorials to learn new skills and gain inspiration.

## 3. Long-Term Commitment

- Focus on Sustainability: The goal of the Primal Plate lifestyle is to create lasting habits that promote health and well-being. Rather than viewing this as a temporary fix, think of it as a lifelong commitment to nourishing your body with wholesome foods.
- Celebrate Progress: Acknowledge and celebrate the small victories along the way—whether it's improved energy levels, better digestion, or simply enjoying cooking more. These positive changes reinforce your commitment and motivate you to continue.
- Connect with Community: Engage with others who share similar values and goals. Whether through online forums, social media groups, or local meet-ups, connecting with like-minded individuals can provide support, inspiration, and encouragement.

As you continue with the Primal Plate lifestyle, remember that you are making powerful choices that lead to better health and well-being. Each decision you make reflects your commitment to nourishing your body and enhancing your quality of life.

You have the strength and resilience to navigate this path with confidence. Every meal you prepare, every new recipe you try, and every mindful choice contributes to your overall health. Celebrate your progress, no matter how small, and recognize that each step forward is a victory.

Let your goals motivate you! Whether you aim to boost your energy levels, improve your fitness, or simply enjoy a more vibrant life, keep that vision at the forefront of your mind. Surround yourself with positivity—seek out supportive communities, share your experiences, and learn from others who share similar values.

Remember that this lifestyle is not about perfection; it's about growth. Allow yourself the flexibility to experiment, adapt, and learn. There will be ups and downs along the way, but each experience provides valuable lessons that help shape your approach to health.

Trust in your ability to make informed choices that align with your health goals. Listen to your body, adjust as needed, and seek out the foods that make you feel your best. With each decision, you reinforce a lifestyle that prioritizes health and vitality.

# Conclusion:

As you reflect on the benefits of a meat-first diet, it's clear that this approach can have transformative effects on your health and wellness. By prioritizing high-quality proteins, you can enhance muscle growth, support recovery, and improve overall energy levels. Additionally, incorporating a variety of nutrient-dense foods alongside your protein sources ensures that you receive essential vitamins and minerals for optimal health.

- Enhanced Muscle Growth: A meat-first diet provides the necessary amino acids to support muscle repair and growth, making it an excellent choice for those looking to increase strength and endurance.
- Improved Energy Levels: Consuming adequate protein helps stabilize blood sugar levels and sustain energy throughout the day, allowing you to perform at your best.
- Better Satiety: High-protein meals can help you feel fuller for longer, reducing cravings and supporting healthy weight management.
- Nutrient Density: Focusing on quality meats and whole foods ensures that you receive a wide range of nutrients that contribute to overall health.

As you continue with this lifestyle, remember that consistency is key. Stay committed to making informed choices that align with your health goals. Embrace the process of learning about nutrition, experimenting with new recipes, and adjusting as needed to find what works best for you.

You have the power to create a fulfilling life centered around health and wellness. Each meal is an opportunity to nourish your body and support your well-being. By making thoughtful choices, you can cultivate a lifestyle that promotes lifelong wellness.

Thank you for taking the time to explore the Primal Plate lifestyle. Your dedication to improving your health is commendable, and I encourage you to continue seeking knowledge and inspiration. For further insights and resources, I invite you to explore my books. They are designed to provide valuable information and guidance on your path to wellness. Together, we can foster a healthier future!